Core Clinical Cases
Problem Based Learning
Self Assessment
for
Medical Students

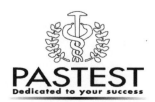

PASTEST
Dedicated to your success

Core Clinical Cases
Problem Based Learning
Self Assessment
for
Medical Students

Andrew Sewart
Final Year Medical Student
University of Liverpool
Liverpool

Henriette van Ruiten
Final Year Medical Student
University of Liverpool
Liverpool

Edited by
Deborah Anne Wales MB ChB MRCP FRCA
Consultant Respiratory Physician
Nevill Hall Hospital
Abergavenny
Monmouthshire

© 2004 PASTEST Ltd
Egerton Court
Parkgate Estate
Knutsford
Cheshire
WA16 8DX

Telephone: 01565 752000

First published 2004

ISBN: 1 904627 358

A catalogue record for this book is available from the British Library.

The information contained within this book was obtained by the authors from
reliable sources. However, while every effort has been made to ensure its
accuracy, no responsibility for loss, damage or injury occasioned to any person
acting or refraining from action as a result of information contained herein can
be accepted by the publishers or authors.

PasTest Revision Books and Intensive Courses
PasTest has been established in the field of postgraduate medical education since
1972, providing revision books and intensive study courses for doctors preparing
for their professional examinations.

Books and courses are available for the following specialties:
MRCGP, MRCP Parts 1 and 2, MRCPCH Parts 1 and 2, MRCPsych, MRCS,
MRCOG Parts 1 and 2, DRCOG, DCH, FRCA, PLAB Parts 1 and 2

For further details contact:
PasTest, Freepost, Knutsford, Cheshire WA16 7BR
Tel: 01565 752000   Fax: 01565 650264
www.pastest.co.uk   enquiries@pastest.co.uk

Text prepared by Carnegie Book Production, Lancaster
Printed and bound by Page Bros (Norwich) Ltd.

DEDICATION

Any similarity between the names of our family and friends and those in the book are purely intentional. However, we wish them all, unlike their namesakes in the book, a long and prosperous life, free of ill health.

We wrote this textbook while as fourth year students based in Lancaster Royal Infirmary. We would like to thank all the staff for their support during the year and we both look forward to working there as junior doctors in a year's time.

CONTRIBUTORS

Dr. Clare Peckham MBBS MRCP 1 MRCPCH DCH
Consultant Paediatrician
Royal Lancaster Infirmary
Lancaster

Dr. Katherine Granger MBBS MRCOG
Consultant Obstetrician and Gynaecologist
Royal Lancaster Infirmary
Lancaster

CONTENTS

FOREWORD

It gave me great pleasure to be asked to review and write the foreword for this book for many reasons . . .

I am delighted that two of our students have been so motivated by their learning that they have wanted to produce a Problem Based Learning book – and stuck with the project through to the end.

I am overjoyed that a book like this has been created – one that takes the problem that the patient presents with and uses that as a focus of learning. Not only is it sensible, as patients do not present with a label round their neck saying 'I have angina' – or 'I have hypothyroidism' – they present with the symptom that as clinicians we have to diagnose and manage, but more importantly, it reminds us that the reason for our learning is not a riddle to be solved but a patient for whose care we are responsible.

As a medical educator I am thrilled that this book has been produced by and for students. It is one of the basic tenets of education that learning is driven by assessment. One of the difficulties about assessment is setting the standard and making it appropriate for the person being assessed – to have that done by and for students helps the student to focus their learning at the right level.

A. S. Garden
Professor of Medical Education
University of Liverpool

INTRODUCTION

In response to the General Medical Council report '*Tomorrow's Doctors*', medical education now puts less emphasis on accumulating factual information and more emphasis on understanding and applying knowledge. At Liverpool (and indeed many other medical schools), medicine is being taught through Problem Based Learning (PBL). For the uninitiated, PBL involves clinical scenarios that students use to formulate their own learning objectives to equip them with the necessary knowledge to manage the patient effectively. We wrote this textbook with PBL in mind. Using clinical scenarios, incorporating more than 60 core clinical cases, a series of questions prompts the reader through the diagnosis, investigations and treatment of each specific case; for added realism, we have also included relevant pharmacology, biochemical and ethical questions as well as the interpretation of X-rays, electrocardiograms and blood results.

We did not just want to write a self-assessment textbook, however. We also wanted to write a concise and practical guide on the management of common cases that would serve as a source of reference during your clinical attachments. For example, we provide information on which tests you should order and, more importantly, why (something we felt is often missing in standard textbooks), so that you are well prepared for even the most fearsome of consultants! We hope we have achieved both aims.

Andrew Sewart **and** Henriette van Ruiten

Lancaster, July 2004.

ABBREVIATIONS

A : C	albumin : creatinine ratio
A&E	Accident and Emergency
ABG	arterial blood gas
ACEI	angiotensin-converting enzyme inhibitor
ALP	alkaline phosphatase
ALT	alanine aminotransferase
AMTS	Abbreviated Mental Test Score
AST	aspartate aminotransferase
BMA	British Medical Association
BNP	B-type or brain natriuretic peptide
BP	blood pressure
CHD	coronary heart disease
CN	cranial nerve
COC	combined oral contraceptive
COPD	chronic obstructive pulmonary disease
COX	cyclo-oxygenase (COX1, COX2)
CPD	cephalo–pelvic disproportion
CPR	cardiopulmonary resuscitation
CTG	cardiotocography
CVD	cardiovascular disease
CVS	cardiovascular system
DC	direct current
DKA	diabetic ketoacidosis
DM	diabetes mellitus
DMARD	disease-modifying antirheumatic drug
DVT	deep vein thrombosis
ECG	electrocardiogram
EPO	erythropoietin
ERCP	endoscopic retrograde cholangiopancreatography
FBC	full blood count
FEV1	forced expiratory volume in 1 s
FVC	forced vital capacity
GI	gastrointestinal
GIFT	gamete intrafallopian transfer
GP	general practitioner

HAV, HBV,	
HCV	hepatitis A, B, and C viruses
HbA1c	glycated haemoglobin
hCG	human chorionic gonadotrophin
HCl	hydrochloric acid
HFEA	Human Fertilisation and Embryology Authority
HIV	human immunodeficiency virus
HPA	hypothalamus–pituitary–adrenal axis
ICP	increased intracranial pressure
ICSI	intracytoplasmic sperm injection
IHD	ischaemic heart disease
im	intramuscular
INR	international normalised ratio
ITU	Intensive Therapy Unit
IUGR	intrauterine growth retardation
iv	intravenous
IVF-ET	in-vitro fertilisation and embryo transfer
KCl	potassium chloride
LAD	left anterior descending
LBBB	left bundle branch block
LFT	liver function test
LVF	left ventricular failure
LVH	left ventricular hypertrophy
MI	myocardial infarction
MMSE	Mini-Mental State Examination
od	once daily
OGD	oesophago-gastro-duodenoscopy
$pCO2$	partial pressure of carbon dioxide
PCOS	polycystic ovarian syndrome
PE	pulmonary embolism
PEFR	peak expiratory flow rate
$pO2$	partial pressure of oxygen
PPI	proton pump inhibitor
PPROM	pre-term pre-labour rupture of membranes
RBBB	right bundle branch block
RSV	respiratory syncytial virus
$saO2$	arterial oxygen saturation
SIADH	syndrome of inappropriate antidiuretic hormone ecretion
SLE	systemic lupus erythematosus

STI	sexually transmitted infection
SUZI	subzonal sperm injection
TC	total cholesterol
TFT	thyroid function test
U&E	urea and electrolytes
UC	ulcerative colitis
USS	ultrasound scan
UTI	urinary tract infection

NORMAL VALUES

Haematology

Haemoglobin	men:	13-18 g/dL
	women:	11.5-16 g/dL
Mean cell volume MCV		76-96 fL
Platelets		150-400 x 109/L
White cells (total)		4-11 x 109/L
INR		0.9-1.2

Arterial blood gases (ABGs)

pH	7.35-7.45
pO2	10-12 kPa
pCO2	4.7-6 kPa
HCO3-	22-28 mmol/L
Base excess	±2 mmol/L

Urea and electrolytes (U&Es)

Sodium	135-145 mmol/L
Potassium	3.5-5 mmol/l
Creatinine	70-120 mmol/l
Urea	2.5-6.7 mmol/L
Albumin	35-50 g/L
Calcium	2.12-2.65 mmol/l
Phosphate	0.8-1.45 mmol/l

Liver function tests (LFTs)

Bilirubin	3-17 µmol/L
Alanine aminotransferase (ALT)	3-35 iu/L
Aspartate transaminase (AST)	3-35 iu/L
Alkaline phosphatase (ALP)	30-150 iu/L
gamma glutamyl transferase (γGT)	11-51 iu/L

Other biochemical values

Amylase	0-180 units/dL
Glucose, fasting	4-6 mmol/L
C-reactive protein (CRP)	<10 mg/L
TSH	0.5-5.7 mu/L
T4 (thyroxine)	70-140 nmol/L
T3 (tri-iodothyroxine)	1.2-3.0 nmol/L

CARDIOVASCULAR CASES: QUESTIONS

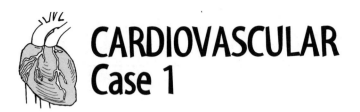

CARDIOVASCULAR
Case 1

Edwin, a 58-year-old KLM pilot, is brought into A&E by ambulance. He has a 45-minute history of central, crushing chest pain associated with nausea, dyspnoea and sweating. On cardiovascular system examination, his blood pressure is 154/96 mmHg, heart rate is 84 bpm and regular; the jugular venous pulse is 4 cm above the sternal angle, the apex beat is not displaced, heart sounds are normal and the chest is clear.

List 6 differential diagnoses   *3 marks*

1.

2.

3.

4.

5.

6.

The ECG is shown:

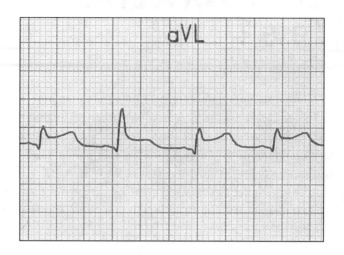

What is the abnormality?   *1 mark*

1.

_____

This abnormality is seen in leads I, aVL and V5/V6.

What is the likely diagnosis?   *2 marks*

1.

_____

What 2 other ECG changes may be expected to develop?   *1 mark*

1.

_____

2.

_____

What 4 brief questions would you ask? *2 marks*

1.

2.

3.

4.

What is your immediate management? *4 marks*

1.

2.

3.

4.

Other than full blood count and urea and electrolytes, what 4 other investigations would you do? *4 marks*

1.

2.

3.

4.

The patient undergoes thrombolysis with streptokinase within 4 hours.

List 2 indications for thrombolysis **2 marks**

1.

2.

Name 3 <u>absolute</u> contraindications for thrombolysis **3 marks**

1.

2.

3.

Edwin is discharged 5 days later with no complications.

What advice, treatment and investigations would you recommend to reduce his risk of a similar episode? **3 marks**

1.

2.

3.

4.

5.

6.

Total: **25 marks**

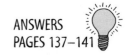

ANSWERS
PAGES 137–141

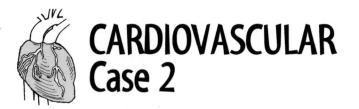

CARDIOVASCULAR
Case 2

Sarah, a 77-year-old retired dog breeder, presents to A&E with a 6-hour history of palpitations and feeling faint. On cardiovascular system examination her heart rate is 120 bpm, blood pressure is 130/90 mmHg; the jugular venous pulse is not raised and the apex beat not displaced; she has a systolic murmur, principally in the 5th intercostal space midclavicular line; the chest is clear.

Her ECG is shown below:

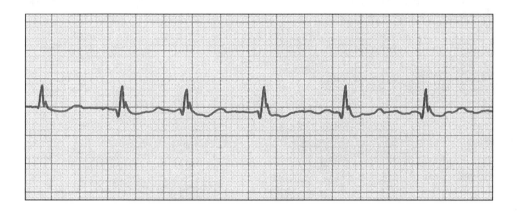

What does the ECG show? **1 mark**

1.

List 4 causes of this rhythm   *2 marks*

1. _____

2. _____

3. _____

4. _____

What is the likely murmur?   *1 mark*

1. _____

What 6 other investigations would you do?   *6 marks*

1. _____

2. _____

3. _____

4. _____

5. _____

6. _____

What 2 drugs may be used to slow down her ventricular rate?   *2 marks*

1. _____

2. _____

Sarah's abnormal rhythm fails to resolve on rate reduction.

What 2 methods may be used to attempt cardioversion?   *2 marks*

1. _____

2. _____

What 3 signs/symptoms would suggest that Sarah is haemodynamically compromised?   *3 marks*

1. _____

2. _____

3. _____

In the event of compromise, what are the first 2 things you should do?   *2 marks*

1. _____

2. _____

Name 3 complications if her abnormal rhythm is not appropriately treated?
     3 marks

1. _____

2. _____

3. _____

What drug is used to prevent embolic events, how is it monitored and what is the target range?   *3 marks*

1.   2.

_____

3.

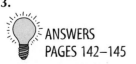
ANSWERS
PAGES 142–145

Total: *25 marks*

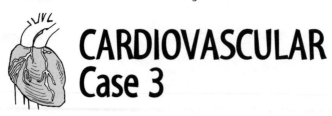

CARDIOVASCULAR
Case 3

Durk, a 54-year-old butcher, has attended his GP for his third blood pressure measurement; his three readings are 167/96, 162/104 and 174/104 mmHg. With regards to his medical history, he is asthmatic and has a body mass index of 28 kg/m².

Define the systolic/diastolic ranges for mild (phase 1), moderate (phase 2) and severe (phase 3) hypertension   *3 marks*

1. Mild:

2. Moderate:

3. Severe:

List 3 causes of secondary hypertension   *3 marks*

1.

2.

3.

What 3 questions would you ask?   *3 marks*

1.

2.

3.

What 6 initial investigations would you do?   *3 marks*

1. _____

2. _____

3. _____

4. _____

5. _____

6. _____

Durk's ECG is shown:

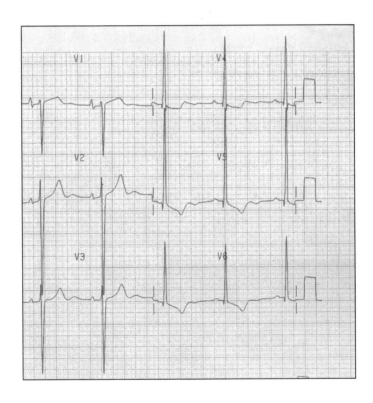

What does his ECG show?   *1 mark*

1.

_____

Would this ECG influence your treatment in someone with hypertension and, if so, why?   *1 mark*

1.

_____

What 3 lifestyle changes would you recommend?   *3 marks*

1.

_____

2.

_____

3.

_____

Name 2 appropriate antihypertensive drugs that may be prescribed to reduce Durk's blood pressure   *2 marks*

1.

_____

2.

_____

Durk is prescribed an angiotensin converting enzyme inhibitor (ACEI) by his GP.

What 2 electrolyte abnormalities may an ACEI cause?   *1 mark*

1.

_____

2.

_____

List 3 circumstances in which you would consider referring a hypertensive patient for specialist care **3 marks**

1.

2.

3.

Name 4 complications if Durk's hypertension is not treated **2 marks**

1.

3.

3.

4.

Total: **25 marks**

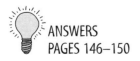

ANSWERS
PAGES 146–150

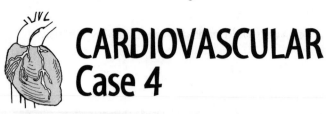

CARDIOVASCULAR
Case 4

Tim, a 60-year-old Professor of Endocrinology, visits his GP complaining of recent episodes of central chest tightness at the end of his golf rounds. These settle on rest and last no longer than 10–15 minutes. There is nothing of note in his past medical history. Cardiovascular examination is normal.

List 5 risk factors you would enquire about in the history   **5 marks**

1.

2.

3.

4.

5.

What 4 initial blood tests would you do and why?   **4 marks**

1.

2.

3.

4.

All these blood tests are normal except a fasting total cholesterol (TC) of 7.2 mmol/l.

What is the recommended upper limit for fasting TC in the secondary prevention of coronary heart disease?   **1 mark**

1.

Tim is prescribed a statin by his GP.

What blood test must you request before prescribing a statin and what advice must you give patients receiving statin therapy?   **2 marks**

1.

2.

Tim's resting ECG is normal. His GP arranges an outpatient appointment for him to undergo an exercise ECG to diagnose angina.

Indicate whether each of the following exercise ECGs represents a negative or positive exercise test   **3 marks**

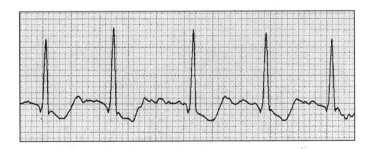

1.

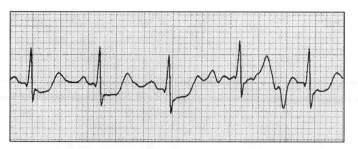

2.

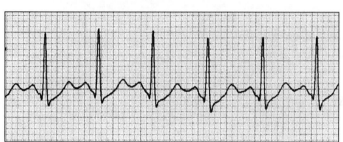

3.

1. ECG 1:

2. ECG 2:

3. ECG 3:

Tim's exercise ECG is positive and a diagnosis of stable angina is made. The cardiologist prescribes aspirin 75 mg od, addresses his modifiable risk factors and places him on the waiting list for coronary angiography.

List 3 drugs that may be prescribed to control angina   **3 marks**

1.

2.

3.

Six months later, Tim undergoes angiography, which shows severe occlusion of the left anterior descending (LAD) artery.

What 2 procedures are available to treat the stenosed LAD?   **2 marks**

1.

2.

Total: **20 marks**

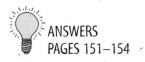

ANSWERS
PAGES 151–154

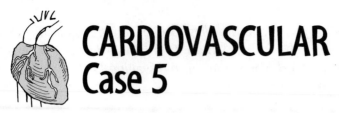

CARDIOVASCULAR
Case 5

Clint, a 72-year-old retired army major, is referred by his GP to the cardiac outpatient department complaining of a 3-month history of progressive breathlessness. He is now breathless even when doing simple tasks around the home, such as ironing. With regards to his past medical history, he is receiving treatment for hypertension and rheumatoid arthritis.

List 4 non-cardiac causes of gradually progressive dyspnoea   ***2 marks***

1.

2.

3.

4.

From the history above, classify his heart failure according to the New York Health Association criteria   ***1 mark***

1.

Cardiovascular

List 4 symptoms suggestive of left ventricular failure (LVF)   *2 marks*

1.

2.

3.

4.

What hormone is significantly increased in heart failure?   *1 mark*

1.

What key investigation would you do to confirm heart failure?   *1 mark*

1.

Clint is diagnosed with left ventricular failure.

Clint's posteroanterior chest X-ray is shown:

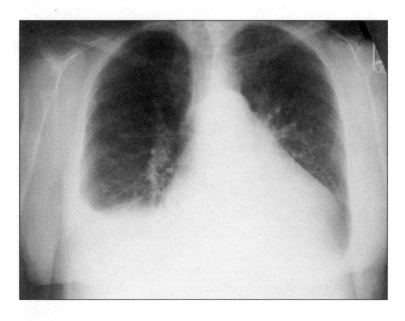

List 4 features seen on Clint's posteroanterior chest X-ray   *2 marks*

1. _____

2. _____

3. _____

4. _____

List 4 causes of LVF   *2 marks*

1. _____

2. _____

3. _____

4. _____

What 3 medications may be exacerbating Clint's LVF?   *3 marks*

1. _____

2. _____

3. _____

Clint is initially prescribed an angiotensin converting enzyme inhibitor (ACEI) and frusemide.

List 3 electrolyte abnormalities caused by frusemide   **3 marks**

1.

2.

3.

Although his frusemide and ACEI therapy is optimised, Clint remains symptomatic, so his cardiologist adds spironolactone and digoxin to his medication.

What electrolyte abnormality potentiates digoxin toxicity?   **1 mark**

1.

What 2 electrolyte abnormalities does digoxin toxicity cause?   **2 marks**

1.

2.

Total: **20 marks**

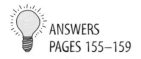

ANSWERS
PAGES 155–159

ENDOCRINOLOGY CASES:
QUESTIONS

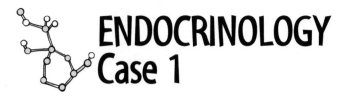

ENDOCRINOLOGY
Case 1

Imke, a 38-year-old child psychologist, is referred by her GP to the endocrinologists; she has symptoms of hyperthyroidism.

Name 6 symptoms Imke may be complaining of   *3 marks*

1.

2.

3.

4.

5.

6.

On examination she is in fast atrial fibrillation, and has a diffuse goitre and bulging eyes.

List 4 signs specific to Graves' disease   *2 marks*

1.

2.

3.

4.

What is the underlying cause of Graves' disease?   **2 marks**

1.

Bloods are taken for thyroid function tests and thyroid-stimulating hormone (TSH) receptor antibodies, confirming the diagnosis of Graves' disease. Her thyroid function test results are shown below.

Indicate (↑, ↓ or →) at '?' the expected changes   **3 marks**

	Normal range	Expected change
TSH	0.5–5.7 munit/l	?
T4	70–140 nmol/l	?
T3	1.2–3.0 nmol/l	?

(TSH = thyroid-stimulating hormone, T3 = tri-iodothyronine, T4 = thyroxine)

Imke is anticoagulated; her symptoms are treated with β-blockers, and her hyperthyroidism by a 'block and replace' regimen with carbimazole and thyroxine.

Give 2 short-term and 2 long-term complications if her hyperthyroidism is untreated   **4 marks**

Short-term complications:

1.

2.

Long-term complications:

1.

2.

Give 4 indications for thyroidectomy in Imke   *2 marks*

1.

2.

3.

4.

Give 4 complications of surgery   *2 marks*

1.

2.

3.

4.

On cessation of the 'block and replace' regimen, Imke remains hyperthyroid. She is subsequently treated with radioactive iodine, which initially renders her euthyroid, though eventually leaves her hypothyroid.

List 4 other causes of hypothyroidism   *2 marks*

1.

2.

3.

4.

Total: *20 marks*

ANSWERS
PAGES 163–167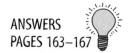

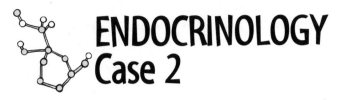

ENDOCRINOLOGY
Case 2

Lysbet, aged 12 years, is seen by her GP after a 3-day history of polyuria, polydipsia, lethargy and recent weight loss, and now complaining of abdominal pain and occasional vomiting. Urine dipstick showed glycosuria and ketonuria and she was admitted to the children's ward. On examination, her Glasgow Coma Scale score is 15/15, her heart rate is 120 bpm; her abdomen is tender throughout, she is hyperventilating and she appears moderately dehydrated.

How is diabetic ketoacidosis (DKA) diagnosed biochemically?   ***3 marks***

1.

2.

3.

Lysbet is diagnosed with DKA. Her venous blood gases are shown below.

Indicate (↑, ↓ or →) at '?' the expected changes   ***3 marks***

	Normal range	**Lysbet's gases**
pH	7.35–7.45	?
pO_2	10–12 kPa	11
pCO_2	4.7–6 kPa	?
HCO_3^-	22–28 mmol/l	?
BE	± 2 mmol/l	-5

(BE = base excess)

Lysbet is successfully treated with iv 0.9% saline and iv insulin.

List 3 complications of this treatment   **3 marks**

1.

2.

3.

List 2 causes of DKA in a child known to have type 1 diabetes   **2 marks**

1.

2.

Once Lysbet's condition has stabilised, she and her parents are seen by the diabetes nurse, who starts her on insulin therapy and educates them on the management of diabetes mellitus.

List 4 'illness rules' you would give Lysbet   **2 marks**

1.

2.

3.

4.

List 4 warning signs of hypoglycaemia   *2 marks*

1.

2.

3.

4.

What 2 co-existing conditions should you screen for in Lysbet?   *2 marks*

1.

2.

How is long-term glycaemic control assessed and what value indicates good control?   *2 marks*

1.

2.

List 4 challenges facing Lysbet and her family   *4 marks*

1.

2.

3.

4.

Lysbet is screened annually to monitor the long-term complications of diabetes mellitus.

List 2 annual screening tests Lysbet should undergo **2 marks**

1.

2.

Total: **25 marks**

ANSWERS
PAGES 168–172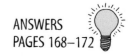

GASTROINTESTINAL CASES:
QUESTIONS

GASTROINTESTINAL
Case 1

George, a 46-year-old known alcoholic, presents to A&E with a 1-hour history of haematemesis, including a severe episode in the ambulance. On examination, his blood pressure is 86/44 mmHg, he is cold peripherally and his pulse is 110 bpm.

What is your immediate management?   ***1 mark***

1.

2.

3.

Which 2 colleagues should you call?   ***1 mark***

1.

2.

List 6 causes of haematemesis   ***3 marks***

1.

2.

3.

continues . . .

4. _____

5. _____

6. _____

What 3 brief questions would you ask? *3 marks*

1. _____

2. _____

3. _____

What 4 blood tests would you request? *2 marks*

1. _____

2. _____

3. _____

4. _____

George's history of chronic alcohol abuse and deranged liver function tests suggested a bleeding oesophageal varice as the cause of his haematemesis. As a result, he underwent emergency endoscopy, confirming a variceal haemorrhage that was successfully treated by injection sclerotherapy and variceal banding.

In patients with oesophageal varices, what drug is used as a prophylaxis against variceal haemorrhage?   *1 mark*

1.

Once his condition is stabilised, George is transferred to the wards for observation.

List 4 signs of a re-bleed while on the ward   *2 marks*

1.

2.

3.

4.

What 2 blood tests may indicate that he has re-bled?   *1 mark*

1.

2.

What 4 questions make up the CAGE questionnaire?   *2 marks*

1. C:

2. A:

3. G:

4. E:

List 2 blood tests to screen for alcohol misuse   *1 mark*

1.

2.

Name 6 other complications of alcohol misuse   *3 marks*

1.

2.

3.

4.

5.

6.

Total: *20 marks*

ANSWERS
PAGES 175–178
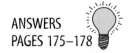

Gastrointestinal

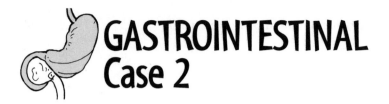

GASTROINTESTINAL
Case 2

Mark, a 44-year-old farmer, visits his GP complaining of a short history of intermittent epigastric pain associated with heartburn and nausea.

List 6 pieces of lifestyle advice to help reduce his dyspepsia   **3 marks**

1.

2.

3.

4.

5.

6.

What drug should be initially prescribed to provide symptomatic relief?   **1 mark**

1.

Mark returns a few weeks later, complaining of a worsening of his symptoms.

List 4 symptoms that would warrant further investigation   *2 marks*

1.

2.

3.

4.

List 6 causes of dysphagia   *3 marks*

1.

2.

3.

4.

5.

6.

List 3 procedures that may be used to investigate his symptoms   *3 marks*

1.

2.

3.

Gastrointestinal

Name 4 complications of gastro-oesophageal reflux disease   **2 marks**

1.

2.

3.

4.

Mark's GP arranges an outpatient appointment for him to undergo upper gastrointestinal endoscopy (oesophago-gastro-duodenoscopy, OGD), which diagnoses oesophagitis.

What drug may be prescribed to treat his oesophagitis?   **1 mark**

1.

In another patient with rheumatoid arthritis receiving long-term non-steroidal anti-inflammatory drug (NSAID) therapy, a gastric ulcer is diagnosed on OGD. The two main causes of peptic ulcer disease are NSAIDs and Helicobacter pylori infection. H. pylori infection is detected by positive serology or ^{13}C-urea breath test and eradicated by a 1-week triple therapy regimen.

What does this regimen involve?   **1 mark**

1.

2.

3.

List 2 other complications of NSAIDs   **1 mark**

1.

2.

Name 2 drugs used to reduce the gastrointestinal side-effects of NSAIDs   **1 mark**

1.

2.

List 4 causes of anaemia in rheumatoid arthritis   **2 marks**

1.

2.

3.

4.

Total: **20 marks**

ANSWERS
PAGES 179–182
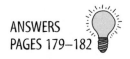

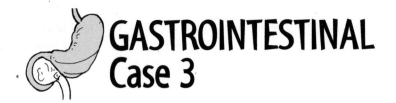

GASTROINTESTINAL
Case 3

Nick, a mountain guide, is admitted to hospital by his GP, complaining of malaise, anorexia and right upper quadrant pain. On examination he is jaundiced and has a palpably enlarged smooth liver and ascites.

List 3 other <u>abdominal</u> signs of liver disease   **3 marks**

1.

2.

3.

List 4 conditions that may cause ascites   **2 marks**

1.

2.

3.

4.

List 4 risk factors for jaundice that you would enquire about in the social history

2 marks

1.

3.

3.

4.

Several blood tests are requested, to assess the severity of Nick's liver disease.

Name 2 blood tests used to assess liver synthetic function   *2 marks*

1.

2.

List 4 extrahepatic causes of the following liver function test profile: aspartate aminotransferase 14 iu/l, alanine aminotransferase 21 iu/l, alkaline phosphatase 270 iu/l, γ-glutamyl transferase (γGT) 77 iu/l, bilirubin 102 μmol/l   *2 marks*

1.

3.

3.

4.

Gastrointestinal

Ultrasound scan reveals an enlarged liver, with hepatic changes consistent with cirrhosis.

In the absence of obvious risk factors, list 3 blood tests you would request to identify the cause of Nick's cirrhosis   **3 marks**

1.

2.

3.

Liver cirrhosis is confirmed by liver biopsy showing micronodular cirrhosis.

What is the most likely cause of Nick's cirrhosis?   **1 mark**

1.

Two days later Nick's condition starts to deteriorate, and he complains of severe abdominal pain. On examination, his abdomen is very tender with guarding and he is pyrexial.

What is the likely complication?   **2 marks**

1.

How would you confirm your diagnosis?   **1 mark**

1.

List 4 other complications of cirrhosis   *2 marks*

1.
_____

2.
_____

3.
_____

4.
_____

Total: *20 marks*

ANSWERS
PAGES 183–187

Gastrointestinal

GASTROINTESTINAL
Case 4

Freda, a 64-year-old lady, presents to A&E with severe sudden-onset right subcostal pain. She also complains of nausea, vomiting and sweating. On examination she has a temperature of 38.4 °C and is tachycardic.

List 6 differential diagnoses   **3 marks**

1.

2.

3.

4.

5.

6.

On examination, you find a positive Murphy's sign.

What is your likely diagnosis?   **1 mark**

1.

Freda's ultrasound scan (USS) is shown:

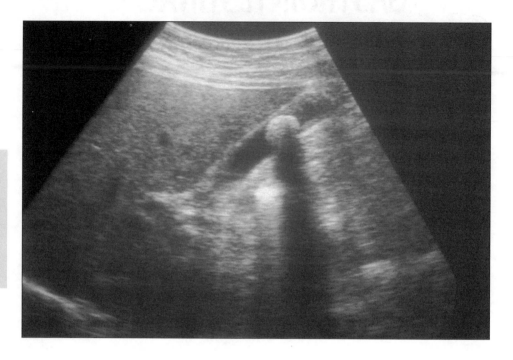

List 4 features on the USS that confirm your diagnosis   ***4 marks***

1.

2.

3.

4.

Freda is initially managed by a nil-by-mouth regimen, iv fluids, antiemetic, im pethidine and prophylactic antibiotics, and she appears to settle on this conservative regimen. She is scheduled for elective cholecystectomy later that week.

Name 6 complications of gallstones   **3 marks**

1.

2.

3.

4.

5.

6.

The next day, however, Freda experiences severe central abdominal pain radiating to her back and vomiting, and appears jaundiced. Her blood test shows an increased serum amylase concentration of 1650 units/dl.

What is the likely complication?   **1 mark**

1.

Name 4 other causes of increased serum amylase   **2 marks**

1.

2.

3.

4.

List 6 blood variables used to assess the severity of her condition   *3 marks*

1. _____

2. _____

3. _____

4. _____

5. _____

6. _____

On examination, Freda shows signs of hypovolaemic shock and is given high-flow O$_2$ and iv saline.

List 6 signs indicating hypovolaemic shock   *3 marks*

1. _____

2. _____

3. _____

4. _____

5. _____

6. _____

In fluid therapy, what minimum urinary output do you aim for?   *1 mark*

1. _____

Give 2 complications of fluid overload **1 mark**

1.

2.

What are the normal daily sodium and potassium requirements? **2 marks**

1.

2.

Freda remains hypotensive despite adequate fluid treatment.

What class of drug would you give Freda? **1 mark**

1.

She is resuscitated on this treatment.

What is the recommended procedure for her condition within the first 72 hours?

1 mark

1.

Freda undergoes a cholecystectomy before discharge.

List 2 advantages each of laparoscopic and open cholecystectomy **2 marks**

1. Laparoscopic:

2. Open:

Give 4 complications of cholecystectomy   *2 marks*

1. _____

2. _____

3. _____

4. _____

Total: *30 marks*

ANSWERS
PAGES 188–194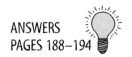

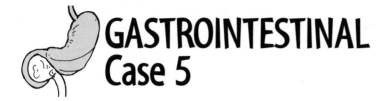

GASTROINTESTINAL
Case 5

Annie, a 25-year-old physiotherapist, presents with a 4-week history of diarrhoea with some mucus and blood mixed in her stool. She also complains of general abdominal discomfort, malaise and weight loss.

List 6 differential diagnoses of weight loss other than malignancy **3 marks**

1.

2.

3.

4.

5.

6.

List 6 causes of bloody diarrhoea   *3 marks*

1. _____

2. _____

3. _____

4. _____

5. _____

6. _____

Why would you do a plain abdominal X-ray in an acute attack of ulcerative
colitis?   *2 marks*

1. _____

*Annie is sent for a sigmoidoscopy, which reveals a superficial
continuous inflammation of the rectum. The mucosa looks
reddened and inflamed, consistent with ulcerative colitis.*

List 3 pathological differences between ulcerative colitis and Crohn's disease
                                                                    3 marks

1. _____

2. _____

3. _____

List 4 extra-intestinal manifestations of inflammatory bowel disease **2 marks**

1. _____

2. _____

3. _____

4. _____

List 6 features used to assess the severity of ulcerative colitis **3 marks**

1. _____

2. _____

3. _____

4. _____

5. _____

6. _____

Annie is treated with oral prednisolone.

Give 8 complications of long-term oral steroid treatment **4 marks**

1. _____

2. _____

3. _____

4. _____

continues . . .

Gastrointestinal

5. _____

6. _____

7. _____

8. _____

What alternative can you prescribe in patients with severe steroid side-effects, to maintain remission and reduce steroid dose? **2 marks**

1. _____

Give 3 complications of inflammatory bowel disease **3 marks**

1. _____

2. _____

3. _____

Total: **25 marks**

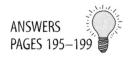

ANSWERS
PAGES 195–199

Gastrointestinal

NEUROLOGICAL CASES: QUESTIONS

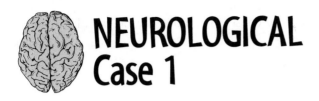 # NEUROLOGICAL
Case 1

Simon, a 72-year-old retired chiropractor, is found collapsed at home with sudden onset hemiparesis without loss of consciousness. Examination reveals signs of an upper motor neurone lesion, sensory loss and homonymous hemianopia on the affected side.

Indicate at '?' the expected findings according to the type of lesion   **4 marks**

	UMN lesion	LMN lesion
Reflexes	?	?
Tone	?	?
Plantars	?	?
Muscle bulk	?	?

(UMN = upper motor neurone, LMN = lower motor neurone)

Name 2 sensory modalities carried in the posterior column   **2 marks**

1.

2.

List 2 visual symptoms Simon might be complaining of   **2 marks**

1.

2.

Neurological

57

Name 4 cardiac conditions that may cause an embolic cerebrovascular accident (CVA) **2 marks**

1.

2.

3.

4.

Simon's brain computed tomography scan is shown:

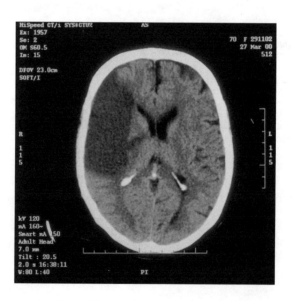

What cerebral artery is affected? **2 marks**

1.

Is Simon's CVA caused by vascular occlusion or haemorrhage? **1 mark**

1.

List 6 features associated with a lesion to the vertebrobasilar territory   *3 marks*

1.

2.

3.

4.

5.

6.

List 6 additional investigations you might consider, briefly explaining why

6 marks

1.

2.

3.

4.

5.

6.

Name 6 health professionals involved in Simon's rehabilitation   *3 marks*

1.

2.

3.

4.

5.

6.

Total: *25 marks*

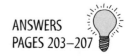

ANSWERS
PAGES 203–207

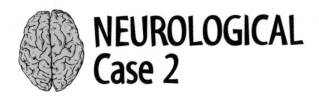

NEUROLOGICAL
Case 2

Mona, an 82-year-old widow, is brought into A&E after her carer found her, that afternoon, still in bed and more confused than normal. On examination she has a Glasgow Coma Scale score of 11/15 and a temperature of 38.5 °C; her blood pressure 116/64 mmHg, her heart rate is 90 bpm and regular; the respiratory rate is 28/min and there is bronchial breathing at her right lung base.

List 6 causes of acute confusion (delirium)   **3 marks**

1.

2.

3.

4.

5.

6.

List 4 non-invasive investigations you would do **2 marks**

1. _____

2. _____

3. _____

4. _____

Mona's blood test results are shown:

Hb	15.1 g/dl	CRP	145 mg/l	pH	7.41
MCV	85 fl			pO_2	7.6 kPa
Platelets	320 x 10⁹/l	Glucose	24.7 mmol/l	pCO_2	5.1 kPa
WCC	21 x 10⁹/l			HCO_3^-	24 mmol/l
	(neutrophilia)	Bilirubin	12 μmol/l		
Na+	149 mmol/l	ALT	14 iu/l	Blood culture Negative	
K+	4.6 mmol/l	AST	12 iu/l		
Urea	28.4 mmol/l	ALP	66 iu/l		
Creatinine	240 mmol/l				

(Hb = haemoglobin, MCV = mean cell volume, WCC = white cell count, CRP = C-reactive protein, ALT = alanine aminotransferase, AST = aspartate aminotransferase, ALP = alkaline phosphatase, pO_2, pCO_2 = partial pressures of oxygen and carbon dioxide, HCO_3^- = bicarbonate)

List 5 diagnoses inferred from these blood results **5 marks**

1. _____

2. _____

3. _____

4. _____

5. _____

List 4 causes of hyponatraemia   **4 marks**

1. _____

2. _____

3. _____

4. _____

A diagnosis of pneumonia is made and Mona is successfully treated with iv cefuroxime and clarithromycin, sliding-scale insulin and iv fluids (0.9% saline). Before she is discharged from hospital, her underlying dementia is assessed and she records a Mini Mental State Examination (MMSE) score of 18.

What MMSE score supports a diagnosis of dementia?   **1 mark**

1. _____

What are the 2 most common causes of dementia?   **1 mark**

1. _____

2. _____

List 4 blood tests you would do to exclude treatable causes of dementia **4 marks**

1. _____

2. _____

3. _____

4. _____

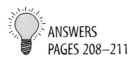
ANSWERS
PAGES 208–211

Total: **20 marks**

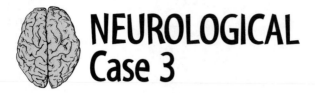 # NEUROLOGICAL
Case 3

While on summer camp in the Brecon Beacons, 17-year-old Meriel is taken ill, complaining of headache, stiff neck and photophobia. Her teachers, worried she may have meningitis, rush her to the nearest A&E department.

Name 2 signs associated with meningeal irritation and briefly describe how they are elicited **2 marks**

1.

2.

A lumbar puncture to confirm the diagnosis is requested and Meriel is examined to exclude increased intracranial pressure (ICP).

List 4 causes of increased ICP **2 marks**

1.

2.

3.

4.

Give 6 signs in Meriel that indicate increased ICP **3 marks**

1.

2. _____

3. _____

4. _____

5. _____

6. _____

Describe what the eye would look like in a complete cranial nerve III palsy

3 marks

1. _____

2. _____

3. _____

Give 2 contraindications (other than increased ICP) to lumbar puncture   *2 marks*

1. _____

2. _____

There are no signs of increased ICP (confirmed on computed tomography scan of the head), and a lumbar puncture is performed.

Indicate (↑, → or ↓) at '?' the expected cerebrospinal fluid (CSF) changes in bacterial meningitis   *2 marks*

Neurological

	Normal	Bacterial meningitis
Appearance	Clear	?
WCC	0–5/mm³	?
Protein	0.2–0.4 g/l	?
Glucose	> 50% of blood glucose	?

(WCC = white cell count)

Meriel is diagnosed with meningococcal meningitis, her CSF Gram staining confirming Neisseria meningitidis.

What colour does *Neisseria meningitidis* give with Gram stain?   *1 mark*

1.

Which antibiotic would you prescribe?   *1 mark*

1.

List 4 complications of bacterial meningitis   *2 marks*

1.

2.

3.

4.

What prophylaxis do you give to contacts of Meriel and what do you warn them about?   *2 marks*

1.

2.

Total: *20 marks*

ANSWERS
PAGES 212–216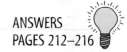

Neurological

OBSTETRICS & GYNAECOLOGY CASES: QUESTIONS

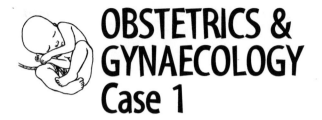

OBSTETRICS & GYNAECOLOGY
Case 1

Sue, a 35-year-old primary school teacher, and her husband Peter, a 38-year-old salesman, are both delighted to discover that Sue is pregnant for the first time. Sue is now 10 weeks pregnant (her last menstrual period was July 15 and her cycle is normally a regular 24 days) and she attends the antenatal clinic for her booking visit.

When is Sue's expected date of delivery?   *1 mark*

1. _____

List 6 blood tests you would offer   *3 marks*

1. _____

2. _____

3. _____

4. _____

5. _____

6. _____

List 4 examples of dietary advice you would give Sue   **2 marks**

1.

2.

3.

4.

List 6 common minor symptoms of pregnancy Sue may experience   **3 marks**

1.

2.

3.

4.

5.

6.

Because of her age, Sue has an increased risk of chromosomal abnormalities, including Down's syndrome (her risk is 1 : 338).

Give an example (including what it measures) of a second trimester screening test for trisomy 21   **2 marks**

1.

Obstetrics & Gynaecology

At 28 weeks, Sue attends the antenatal clinic complaining of feeling tired and having fainted 2 days previously.

What 2 conditions should you exclude?   *1 mark*

1.

2.

How do you screen for pre-eclampsia   *1 mark*

1.

List 4 symptoms associated with pre-eclampsia   *2 marks*

1.

2.

3.

4.

On obstetric examination, the midwife finds that the pubic symphysis (fundal) height is 24 cm.

Give 4 reasons why Sue may be small for dates   *2 marks*

1.

2.

3.

4.

List 4 causes of intrauterine growth retardation   **4 marks**

1.

2.

3.

4.

List 4 topics you want to discuss with Sue in her third trimester   **4 marks**

1.

2.

3.

4.

Total: **25 marks**

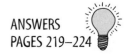

ANSWERS
PAGES 219–224

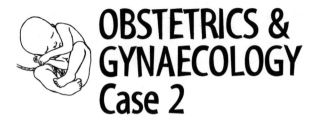

OBSTETRICS & GYNAECOLOGY Case 2

26-year-old Debbie, 39 weeks pregnant with her first child, is out walking when her waters break. She is rushed to the labour ward by her husband Gerald and is complaining of regular painful contractions every 10 minutes.

List 4 questions you would ask   **2 marks**

1.

2.

3.

4.

On obstetric palpation, fundal height is 40 cm, it is a cephalic presentation and the fetal head is engaged. On vaginal examination, the position is left occiput-lateral and the cervix is 4 cm dilated.

List 6 <u>maternal</u> observations recorded on the partogram   *3 marks*

1. _____

2. _____

3. _____

4. _____

5. _____

6. _____

Debbie's contractions become progressively more frequent and painful. Three hours later her cervical dilatation is reassessed and plotted on the partogram, demonstrating that Debbie's labour is progressing satisfactorily.

Give 2 examples each of non-pharmacological and pharmacological methods of pain relief   *2 marks*

1. Non-pharmacological: _____

2. Pharmacological: _____

By how many centimetres should the cervix be dilated now?   *1 mark*

1. _____

List 4 causes of failure to progress in the first stage of labour   **2 marks**

1.

2.

3.

4.

During labour, Debbie's baby is intermittently monitored by cardiotocography (CTG) to assess whether her baby is distressed.

What 4 components are used to interpret a CTG?   **2 marks**

1.

2.

3.

4.

List 4 sequential stages in the passage of the fetus through the birth canal leading up to the delivery of the shoulders   **4 marks**

1.

3.

3.

4.

Debbie delivers a pink and healthy boy, named Alex, who cries immediately.

List 4 steps in your immediate management of Alex **2 marks**

1.

2.

3.

4.

As Alex is born, Debbie is given im oxytocin. After birth, the placenta is removed by controlled cord traction and inspected for completeness.

Give 2 non-pharmacological techniques for reducing postpartum haemorrhage **1 mark**

1.

2.

Name 2 drugs that are used to reduce postpartum haemorrhage **1 mark**

1.

2.

Total: **20 marks**

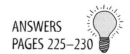

ANSWERS
PAGES 225–230

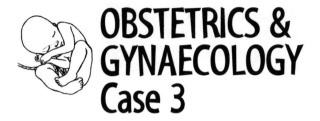

OBSTETRICS & GYNAECOLOGY
Case 3

Katie, who is 28 weeks into her first pregnancy, suddenly experiences a gush of fluid vaginally in the absence of any uterine contractions. Cardiotocography is normal and ultrasound scan shows residual amniotic fluid. A speculum examination is performed, which reveals a closed cervix and pooling of fluid in the posterior fornix.

List 4 causes of pre-term pre-labour rupture of membranes (PPROM)   ***2 marks***

1.

2.

3.

4.

What common vaginal organism is Katie's baby at risk from?   ***1 mark***

1.

List 2 treatments to minimise perinatal complications   ***2 marks***

1.

2.

On examination, Katie's temperature is 38 °C, her heart rate is 92 bpm and she has increased white cell count and C-reactive protein. In view of the risks of maternal and fetal infection, it is decided to induce labour. Her cervix is assessed using the Bishop's score.

List 4 features used to assess the Bishop's score   **2 marks**

1.

2.

3.

4.

What Bishop's score is considered ripe for induction?   **1 mark**

1.

What is used to make the cervix ripe for induction?   **1 mark**

1.

Katie's contractions are inefficient, so she is started with an infusion of oxytocin.

List 2 potential complications of using oxytocin in Katie   **2 marks**

1.

2.

Katie delivers a girl, Jacoba, weighing 1.1 kg. At 1 minute of life, Jacoba's extremities are blueish, her limbs flaccid, her breathing is irregular, she grimaces when the soles of her feet are stimulated and her heart rate is 82 bpm.

Calculate Jacoba's 1-minute Apgar score   **2 marks**

1.

Within an hour of birth, Jacoba starts developing signs of respiratory distress. Her trachea is intubated by the neonatologist, artifical surfactant is instilled and her lungs are ventilated by continuous positive airways pressure.

List 4 pulmonary causes of respiratory distress in a neonate   **2 marks**

1.

2.

3.

4.

List 2 complications of artificially ventilating Jacoba's lungs   **2 marks**

1.

2.

3.

4.

Jacoba's chest X-ray is shown:

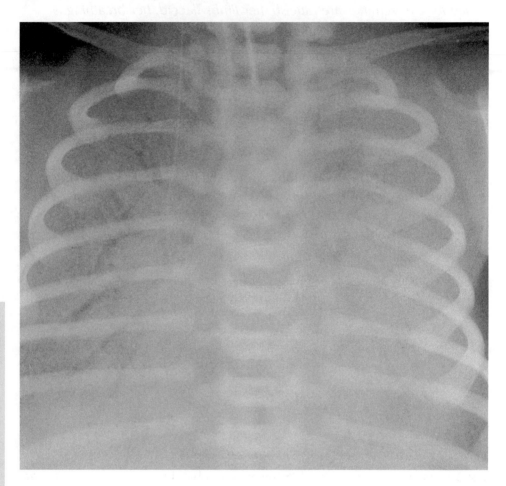

Describe 3 abnormalities on the chest X-ray   *3 marks*

1.

2.

3.

Total: **20 marks**

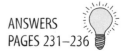

ANSWERS
PAGES 231–236

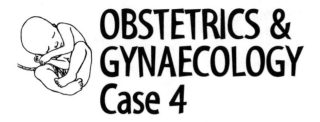

OBSTETRICS & GYNAECOLOGY Case 4

Paul and Julie (both aged 33 years) visit their GP after 2 years of being unable to conceive. A full history is taken from both. Julie's gynaecological history reveals irregular periods.

List 4 points in a full history suggestive of tubal dysfunction **2 marks**

1.

2.

3.

4.

The GP organises semen analysis for Paul and an outpatient hysterosalpingogram to assess tubal patency in Julie, and requests a number of blood tests.

List 4 variables measured in semen analysis **2 marks**

1.

2.

3.

4.

The results come back confirming normal semen analysis, and patent tubes. Julie's blood results are shown:

Haemoglobin	12 g/dl (normal range 11.5–16 g/dl)
Rubella	Seronegative
Rhesus	Positive
LH (day 2)	18 units/l (normal range 3–16 units/l)
FSH (day 2)	6 units/l (normal range 2–8 units/l)
Progesterone (day 21)	18 nmol/l

(LH = luteinising hormone, FSH = follicle-stimulating hormone)

What is a normal day-21 progesterone concentration?   *1 mark*

1.

Give 2 explanations for Julie's progesterone concentration   *2 marks*

1.

2.

What might a day-2 FSH much greater than 10 units/l suggest?   *1 mark*

1.

What is your likely diagnosis?   *1 mark*

1.

List 3 clinical features which Julie might have   **3 marks**

1.

2.

3.

Julie is referred to her local infertility clinic, where her infertility is treated with clomiphene.

List 3 complications associated with this treatment   **3 marks**

1.

2.

3.

List 2 treatments Julie should be offered before conception   **2 marks**

1.

2.

What do IVF-ET, ICSI, GIFT and SUZI stand for?   *2 marks*

1. IVF-ET:

2. ICSI:

3. GIFT:

4. SUZI:

What is the name of the organisation that regulates all assisted conception treatments?   *1 mark*

1.

Total: *20 marks*

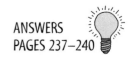

ANSWERS
PAGES 237–240

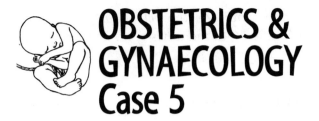

OBSTETRICS & GYNAECOLOGY Case 5

Ageeth, a 26-year-old personal assistant, visits her GP requesting the pill because her new boyfriend doesn't like using condoms.

Describe 3 contraceptive mechanisms of the combined oral contraceptive (COC)

3 marks

1.

2.

3.

List 6 contraindications to the COC **6 marks**

1.

2.

3.

4.

5.

6.

Nothing in Ageeth's history contraindicates the pill. She is prescribed a 3-month supply of a COC and advised on its side-effects.

Name 6 <u>minor</u> side effects Ageeth may experience   **3 marks**

1.

2.

3.

4.

5.

6.

List 6 pieces of additional advice you would give Ageeth   **3 marks**

1.

2.

3.

4.

5.

6.

Several months later, Ageeth attends her genitourinary medicine clinic complaining of an offensive vaginal discharge.

List 4 additional clinical features that would suggest pelvic inflammatory disease

2 marks

1.

2.

3.

4.

What 6 questions would you ask in the sexual history?   **3 marks**

1.

2.

3.

4.

5.

6.

List 4 infective causes of vaginal discharge   **2 marks**

1.

2.

3.

4.

Endocervical and high vaginal swabs are taken. Microscopy reveals pink Gram-stained diplococci.

What is the likely cause of her vaginal discharge?   **1 mark**

1.

List 4 additional tests you would offer Ageeth   **2 marks**

1.

2.

3.

4.

Total: **25 marks**

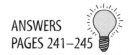

ANSWERS
PAGES 241–245

Obstetrics & Gynaecology

PAEDIATRIC CASES:
QUESTIONS

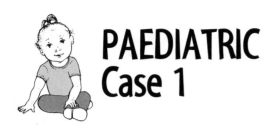

PAEDIATRIC
Case 1

Jim, aged 18 months, is referred to the paediatric outpatient clinic because of poor weight gain over the past 6 months. Apart from two admissions to hospital for bronchiolitis in his first year of life, he was a thriving and happy infant. However, over the past 6 months his mother says he has become irritable, his abdomen seems distended and he has lots of liquid stools, which are foul smelling and difficult to flush. On examination, Jim is pale and his abdomen is protruded. There is wasting of his muscles (especially buttocks) and his ankles seem swollen.

Define failure to thrive   **2 marks**

1. _____

List 2 causes for weight below the 0.4th centile other than failure to thrive
                                                                                 2 marks

1. _____

2. _____

List 3 non-organic causes of failure to thrive   **3 marks**

1. _____

2. _____

3. _____

What is the cause of Jim's diarrhoea?   *1 mark*

1.

___

What is the underlying cause of Jim's ankle oedema?   *1 mark*

1.

___

As part of his investigations, Jim is screened for cystic fibrosis and coeliac disease.

Briefly outline the cause of diarrhoea in cystic fibrosis and coeliac disease

2 marks

1. Cystic fibrosis:

2. Coeliac disease:

___

List 2 causes of failure to thrive in cystic fibrosis   *2 marks*

1.

2.

___

What test do you use to screen for cystic fibrosis and what represents a positive result?   *1 mark*

1.

2.

Jim's cystic fibrosis screen is negative, but the coeliac disease screen comes back as positive for anti-gliadin and anti-endomysial antibodies. He then undergoes a jejunal biopsy, which histologically confirms coeliac disease.

List 2 jejunal histological changes seen in coeliac disease   *1 mark*

1. _____

2. _____

How else may coeliac disease present?   *1 mark*

1. _____

List 3 food groups Jim will now have to avoid   *3 marks*

1. _____

2. _____

3. _____

Jim is put on a gluten-free diet and within 2 months he has caught up on his growth and is back to his usually happy self. His mother asks whether the diagnosis of coeliac disease is for life?

What do you tell Jim's mother?   *1 mark*

1. _____

Total: *20 marks*

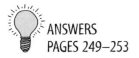
ANSWERS
PAGES 249–253

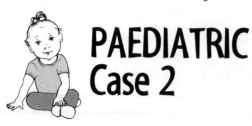

PAEDIATRIC
Case 2

Baby Rebecca is born at 40 weeks gestation, by normal vaginal delivery and weighing 3.2 kg. Her mother (gravida 1, para 1) went into labour spontaneously and labour was not prolonged. Rebecca's Apgar scores were 9 and 10 at 1 and 5 minutes, respectively, and she was transferred to the postnatal ward together with her mother. At the postnatal check the next day, the midwife notices that Rebecca's skin and sclera are yellow. Apart from that she appears very well and is breast-feeding satisfactorily.

Are you concerned about Rebecca's jaundice? Briefly explain your reasoning?

2 marks

1.

2.

Give 3 reasons why jaundice is common in neonates   *3 marks*

1.

2.

3.

Paediatric

Rebecca's jaundice is investigated. Her blood results are shown:

Haemoglobin	12.2 g/dl (normal range 14.5–21.5 g/dl)
Platelets	220 x 10⁹/l (normal range 150–400 x 10⁹/l)
MCV	112 fl (normal range 100–135 fl)
WCC	14 x 10⁹/l (normal range 10–26 x 10⁹/l)
Total serum bilirubin	140 µmol/l (normal range 3–17 µmol/l) (unconjugated)
CRP	< 10 mg/l
Film	Normal RBCs
Rebecca's blood group	A, Rh -ve
Maternal blood group	O, Rh -ve
Direct Coombs' Test	+ (mildly +ve)

(MCV = mean cell volume, WCC = white cell count, CRP = C-reactive protein, RBC = red blood cell, Rh -ve = Rhesus-negative, +ve = positive)

Give 3 causes of increased <u>conjugated</u> bilirubin in neonates   *3 marks*

1.

2.

3.

What does the direct Coombs' test detect, and what does it indicate?   *2 marks*

1.

2.

From the blood results, what is the cause of Rebecca's jaundice?   *2 marks*

1.

What is your initial management?   *1 mark*

1. _____

Because bilirubin concentrations are increasing (second measurement showed a bilirubin concentration of 280 μmol/l), phototherapy is started.

How does phototherapy work?   *1 mark*

1. _____

If unconjugated bilirubin reaches high concentrations (> 360 μmol/l) it can become neurotoxic. This happens when bilirubin concentrations exceed the binding capacity of albumin, allowing unbound unconjugated bilirubin to cross the blood–brain barrier.

What is this neurotoxicity called?   *1 mark*

1. _____

Give 3 signs of this   *3 marks*

1. _____

2. _____

3. _____

Give 2 long-term complications of this **2 marks**

1.

2.

Fortunately for Rebecca, phototherapy is successful and she joins her new family at home 4 days later, receiving oral folic acid. She is followed up as an outpatient 2 weeks later for a repeat full blood count, to ensure late haemolysis is not occurring.

Total: **20 marks**

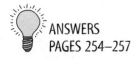

ANSWERS
PAGES 254–257

Paediatric

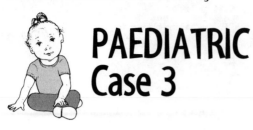

PAEDIATRIC
Case 3

Erik, aged 8 months, is brought into A&E by his parents 6 days before Christmas, with a 2-day history of feeding difficulties preceded by coryzal symptoms. On examination, his temperature is 38.5 °C, he is mildly dehydrated and tachycardic, and has signs of respiratory distress, with a widespread expiratory wheeze; his saO_2 (on air) is 90%.

List 6 signs of respiratory distress in an infant   **3 marks**

1.

2.

3.

4.

5.

6.

What are the normal heart rate and respiratory rate in infants?   **2 marks**

1. Heart rate (bpm):

2. Respiratory rate (/min):

Paediatric

List 6 investigations involved in a septic screen   *3 marks*

1.

2.

3.

4.

5.

6.

List 4 signs indicating dehydration in an infant   *2 marks*

1.

2.

3.

4.

A diagnosis of bronchiolitis is made and Erik is cohorted on the ward and barrier-nursed to prevent spread of virus.

List 4 types of paediatric patients at risk of bronchiolitis   *2 marks*

1.

2.

3.

4.

What is the common cause of bronchiolitis and how is it detected?   *2 marks*

1.

2.

How would you manage Erik?   *4 marks*

1.

2.

3.

4.

How would you monitor the effectiveness of treatment?   *2 marks*

1.

2.

3.

4.

Total: *20 marks*

ANSWERS
PAGES 258–261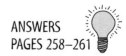

Paediatric

RESPIRATORY CASES:
QUESTIONS

RESPIRATORY
Case 1

Lucy, a 21-year-old asthmatic, presents to A&E with a 2-day history of increased shortness of breath, wheeze and cough. On examination, her temperature is 37.9 °C, her pulse is 125 bpm and her blood pressure 130/80 mmHg; respiratory rate is 30/min, there is widespread bilateral expiratory wheeze and air entry is reduced throughout.

List 3 criteria used to indicate a severe asthma attack   ***3 marks***

1.

2.

3.

List 6 criteria used to indicate a life-threatening asthma attack   ***3 marks***

1.

2.

3.

4.

5.

6.

What is your immediate management in severe asthma?   **3 marks**

1.

2.

3.

What are the 2 indications for iv aminophylline?   **1 mark**

1.

2.

What 3 brief questions would you ask?   **3 marks**

1.

2.

3.

What 4 blood tests would you do?   **2 marks**

1.

2.

3.

4.

Give 2 reasons why you would request a chest X-ray   *1 mark*

1.

2.

The arterial blood gas results (on air) are shown:

pH   7.31 (normal range 7.35–7.45)

pO_2 7.7 kPa (normal range 10–12 kPa)

pCO_2 3.4 kPa (normal range 4.7–6 kPa)

HCO_3^- 16 mmol/l (normal range 22–28 mmol/l)

What do these results indicate?   *1 mark*

1.

List 2 ways in which the effects of treatment can be assessed non-invasively

1 mark

1.

2.

Lucy's breathing improves and she is transferred to the wards.

What 4 things should Lucy have before discharge?   *2 marks*

1.

2.

3.

4.

Total: *20 marks*

ANSWERS
PAGES 265–268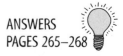

Respiratory

RESPIRATORY
Case 2

Tom, a 73-year-old lifelong smoker with known chronic obstructive pulmonary disease (COPD), is brought into A&E with severe dyspnoea and cough productive of green sputum. On examination, his temperature is 38 °C and his pulse is 95 bpm; his respiratory rate is 35/min, he has widespread expiratory wheeze, reduced air entry throughout and is cyanosed.

List 4 differential diagnoses   *2 marks*

1.

2.

3.

4.

What 4 brief questions would you ask regarding his COPD?   *2 marks*

1.

2.

3.

4.

What is your immediate management?   *3 marks*

1. _____

2. _____

3. _____

What 4 blood tests would you do?   *2 marks*

1. _____

2. _____

3. _____

4. _____

What 4 non-invasive investigations would you do?   *2 marks*

1. _____

2. _____

3. _____

4. _____

The arterial blood gas results (on air) are shown:

pH   7.37 (normal range 7.35–7.45)

pO_2 6.9 kPa (normal range 10–12kPa)

pCO_2 4.2 kPa (normal range 4.7–6 kPa)

HCO_3^- 25 mmol/l (normal range 22–28 mmol/l)

What do the arterial blood gases indicate?   **2 marks**

1.

_____

How will these results influence your immediate management?   **1 mark**

1.

_____

List 4 signs of hypercapnia   **2 marks**

1.

_____

2.

_____

3.

_____

4.

_____

From his past medical history, Tom is considered at high risk of cardiopulmonary arrest. He informs you of an advance directive refusing cardiopulmonary resuscitation (CPR).

List 4 forms in which an advance directive can be made   **2 marks**

1.

_____

2.

_____

3.

_____

4.

_____

Respiratory

Name 2 of Tom's human rights broken if CPR were to be performed   *2 marks*

1. _____

2. _____

The diagnosis of exacerbation of infective COPD is made; this is successfully treated with amoxicillin.

What 2 organisms are commonly responsible for COPD exacerbations?   *1 mark*

1.   _____

2.   _____

List 4 issues to be addressed on discharge, in collaboration with Tom's GP

2 marks

1. _____

2. _____

3. _____

4. _____

List 2 qualifying criteria for home O_2 therapy   *2 marks*

1. _____

2. _____

Total: *25 marks*

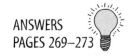

ANSWERS
PAGES 269–273

RESPIRATORY
Case 3

Charlotte, a 30-year-old secretary, presents to A&E with sudden onset of severe right-sided chest pain exacerbated by inspiration, with associated breathlessness and feeling dizzy. She is normally fit and well, having recently returned from a week's holiday in Florida with her boyfriend. She is not taking any prescribed medicines except the combined oral contraceptive pill. The abnormal findings on examination are: heart rate 104 bpm, respiratory rate 22/min and a tender, swollen right calf.

List 6 risk factors for pulmonary embolism   **3 marks**

1.

2.

3.

4.

5.

6.

List 3 differential diagnoses for a tender, swollen calf   **3 marks**

1.

2.

3.

Respiratory

What is your immediate management?   *2 marks*

1.

2.

3.

4.

What 6 investigations would you do?   *6 marks*

1.

2.

3.

4.

5.

6.

Charlotte's ECG is shown:

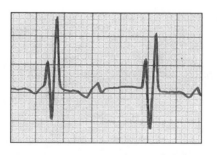

(VI trace shown)

What does this ECG show? **1 mark**

1. _____

The diagnosis of pulmonary embolism secondary to a deep vein thrombosis (DVT) is made. Charlotte is discharged on a 6-month course of warfarin with a target international normalised ratio (INR) of 2–3 and an anticoagulant card to carry.

What 4 pieces of general advice would you give to prevent a DVT during a plane flight? **2 marks**

1. _____

2. _____

3. _____

4. _____

Six weeks later, Charlotte is treated by her GP with erythromycin (an enzyme inhibitor), for a minor chest infection.

Is she at risk, if so of what and how should this be assessed? **3 marks**

1. _____

2. _____

3. _____

Total: **20 marks**

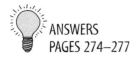

ANSWERS
PAGES 274–277

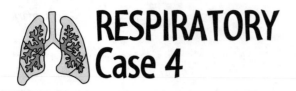

RESPIRATORY
Case 4

*Debbie, a 64-year-old heavy smoker, visits her GP complaining of a
3-month history of cough associated with haemoptysis.*

List 3 respiratory causes of haemoptysis   ***3 marks***

1.

2.

3.

List 2 other common presenting symptoms of lung cancer   ***2 marks***

1.

2.

*On examination, the only abnormal finding is that she has clubbing
of the fingers.*

List 2 cardiac, 2 respiratory and 2 gastrointestinal causes of clubbing   ***3 marks***

1. Cardiac:

2. Gastrointestinal:

3. Respiratory:

The GP arranges an urgent chest X-ray. The radiological report notes opacification of the right apex, with destruction of the second rib, consistent with bronchial carcinoma.

Debbie's chest X-ray is shown:

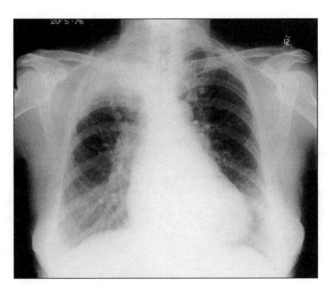

What is this type of lung tumour called?   *1 mark*

1.

List 4 signs of Horner's syndrome   *2 marks*

1.

2.

3.

4.

List 4 causes of round lesions on the lung on chest X-ray **2 marks**

1. _____

2. _____

3. _____

4. _____

Debbie is seen the following week as an outpatient at the respiratory clinic.

List 3 blood tests you would request **3 marks**

1. _____

2. _____

3. _____

What 2 investigations would you arrange to confirm lung cancer? **2 marks**

1. _____

2. _____

From these tests a diagnosis of inoperable squamous cell bronchial carcinoma is confirmed. Three months later, Debbie is admitted with unremitting back pain causing night-time waking. A lateral spinal X-ray confirms secondary deposits in the thoracic vertebrae. She is treated with radiotherapy and opioid analgesia. The bone profile results are shown:

Bone Profile Results

Ca^{2+}	3.7 mmol/l (normal range 2.12–2.65 mmol/l)
$(PO_4)^{3-}$	1.4 mmol/l (normal range 0.8–1.45 mmol/l)
ALP	190 iu (normal range 30–150 iu)
$((PO_4)^{3-}=$	phosphate, ALP = alkaline phosphatase)

List 5 causes of increased serum calcium   **5 marks**

1.

2.

3.

4.

5.

How would you reduce Debbie's serum calcium?   **2 marks**

1.

2.

Total: **25 marks**

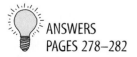

ANSWERS
PAGES 278–282

RESPIRATORY
Case 5

John, a 63-year-old diabetic carpenter, attends his GP with a 3-day history of cough productive of green sputum, pyrexia and general malaise. He is prescribed amoxicillin, but continues to deteriorate and is admitted to hospital the following day.

John's chest X-ray is shown:

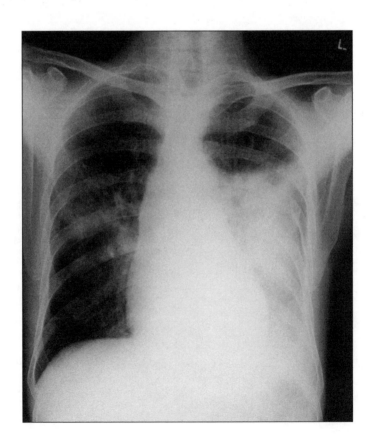

What is your diagnosis?   *1 mark*

1.

List 2 poor prognostic features in the history above   *2 marks*

1.

2.

A full examination is performed and blood taken for full blood count, urea and electrolytes, C-reactive protein (CRP), arterial blood gases, liver function tests, glucose and culture.

List 3 findings on <u>examination</u> that would indicate severe pneumonia   *3 marks*

1.

2.

3.

List 3 findings on <u>investigation</u> that would indicate severe pneumonia   *3 marks*

1.

2.

3.

Respiratory

John is treated with O_2 to maintain his arterial oxygen saturation (saO_2) > 92%, paracetamol for his pleuritic chest pain and oral antibiotics (amoxicillin and erythromycin, to cover atypical organisms).

List 3 causes of 'atypical' pneumonia **3 marks**

1.

2.

3.

List 6 parameters used to assess the progress of treatment **3 marks**

1.

2.

3.

4.

5.

6.

John's blood results are shown:

Hb	13.1 g/dl	CRP	267 mg/l	pH	7.39
MCV	85 fl			pO_2	9.1 kPa
Platelets	320 x 10⁹/l	Glucose	8.2 mmol/l	pCO_2	4.9 kPa
WCC	14 x 10⁹/l			HCO_3^-	24 mmol/l
		Bilirubin	11 µmol/l		
Na⁺	141 mmol/l	ALT	17 iu/l	Blood culture	Gram +ve cocci
K⁺	4.6 mmol/l	AST	14 iu/l		
Urea	6.1 mmol/l	ALP	54 iu/l		
Creatinine	112 mmol/l				

(Hb = haemoglobin, MCV = mean cell volume, WCC = white cell count, CRP = C-reactive protein, ALT = alanine aminotransferase, AST = aspartate aminotransferase, ALP = alkaline phosphatase, pO_2, pCO_2 = partial pressures of oxygen and carbon dioxide, HCO_3^- = bicarbonate)

What is the most likely cause of John's pneumonia, and how can this be prevented? *2 marks*

1.

2.

John's temperature and CRP remain high and clinical examination reveals reduced breath sounds at the right base. His chest X-ray is repeated (and shows a right pleural effusion).

What is the most likely complication? *1 mark*

1.

How should this be treated?   *2 marks*

1.

2.

Total: *20 marks*

ANSWERS
PAGES 283–287

RHEUMATOLOGY CASES: QUESTIONS

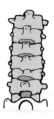 # RHEUMATOLOGY
Case 1

Kristine, a 36-year-old nurse, is referred to the Rheumatology outpatient department with a 2-month history of stiff, painful, swollen hands associated with general malaise.

List 4 inflammatory causes of polyarthropathy **4 marks**

1.

2.

3.

4.

Examination of Kristine's hands and wrists shows changes characteristic of rheumatoid arthritis (RA).

Give 8 features of RA in the hands and wrists on examination **4 marks**

1.

2.

3.

4

5.

6. _____

7. _____

8. _____

Kristine is sent for an X-ray of her hands.

Give 4 X-ray changes in the hands in RA   **2 marks**

1. _____

2. _____

3. _____

4. _____

List 4 criteria on history, examination and investigation used to diagnose RA in Kristine   **4 marks**

1. _____

2. _____

3. _____

4. _____

List 4 features associated with a poor prognosis **2 marks**

1. _____

2. _____

3. _____

4. _____

Kristine is diagnosed with RA and initially treated with non-steroidal anti-inflammatory drugs. However, because of pain and progressive loss of function, her rheumatologist prescribes a disease-modifying antirheumatic drug (DMARD).

Name 2 DMARDs and 2 side-effects associated with each **4 marks**

DMARD	Associated side-effects
1.	1.
	2.
2.	1.
	2.

(DMARD = disease-modifying antirheumatic drug)

Total: 20 marks

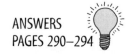
ANSWERS
PAGES 290–294

Rheumatology

UROLOGICAL CASES:
QUESTIONS

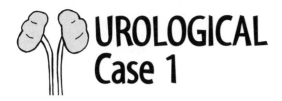

UROLOGICAL
Case 1

Rommy, a 49-year-old busy housewife, is investigated for malaise and fatigue by her GP. Her current medications are insulin, angiotensin converting enzyme inhibitor (for hypertension) and non-steroidal anti-inflammatory drug (for chronic back pain). Her blood results are shown:

Hb	9.2 g/dl	Na+	136 mmol/l
MCV	86 fl	K+	5.7 mmol/l
WCC	5.2 x 10⁹/l	Urea	27 mmol/l
Platelets	280 x 10⁹/l	Creatinine	195 μmol/l
Glucose	18.7 mmol/l	Ca²⁺	1.82 mmol/l
HbA1c	9.2%	(PO₄)³⁻	2.72 mmol/l

(Hb = haemoglobin, MCV = mean cell volume, WCC = white cell count, HbA1c = glycated haemoglobin, $(PO_4)^{3-}$ = phosphate)

List 3 blood tests suggestive of chronic renal failure **3 marks**

1.

2.

3.

What is the likely cause of her anaemia? **1 mark**

1.

Name 4 factors that might be contributing to Rommy's renal failure   *2 marks*

1. _____

2. _____

3. _____

4. _____

List 4 <u>systemic</u> causes of pruritus   *2 marks*

1. _____

2. _____

3. _____

4. _____

*Rommy is referred to a nephrologist for her chronic renal failure
and is kept under review for progression of her disease and to
prevent or treat any complications.*

List 2 treatments to prevent renal bone disease   *2 marks*

1. _____

2. _____

How would you monitor the effectiveness of such treatment?   *1 mark*

1. _____

A graph of Rommy's reciprocal plasma creatinine concentration against time is shown:

RENAL FUNCTION

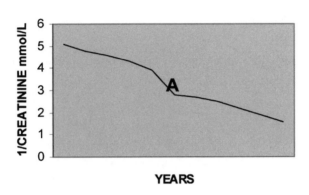

Give 4 possible causes for the sharp decline at time A   *2 marks*

1.

2.

3.

4.

Rommy is referred for haemodialysis when her plasma creatinine reaches 650 μmol/l and is put on the waiting list for renal transplantation.

List 3 other indications for dialysis in chronic renal failure **3 marks**

1. _____

2. _____

3. _____

Give 2 arguments for and 2 arguments against commercial kidney donation

4 marks

For: _____

1. _____

2. _____

Against: _____

1. _____

2. _____

Total: **20 marks**

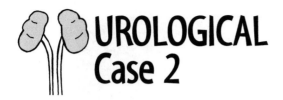

UROLOGICAL
Case 2

Friso, a 39-year-old managing director, presents to A&E with severe left-sided loin pain radiating down to his groin; he also complains of vomiting and sweating.

List 3 urine chemical abnormalities predisposing to urinary stone formation

3 marks

1.

2.

3.

List 2 findings on urine dipstick suggestive of a urinary tract infection **1 mark**

1.

2.

Name 2 bacterial causes of urinary tract infection **1 mark**

1.

2.

Friso's film is shown, demonstrating a dilated left renal pelvis, clubbed calyces and ureteric obstruction:

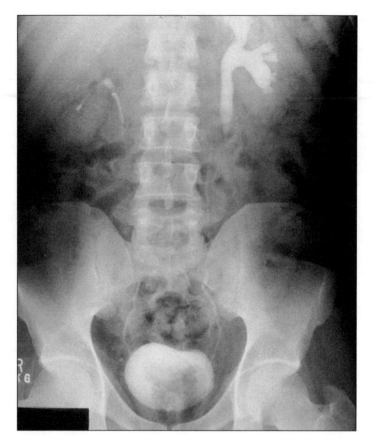

What is the name of this investigation? **1 mark**

1.
_____

Friso's urea and electrolyte data indicate acute renal failure with hyperkalaemia.

List 2 causes each of pre-renal, renal-renal and post-renal failure **6 marks**

Pre-renal:
_____

1.
_____

2.
_____

Renal-renal:

1.

2.

Post-renal:

1.

2.

List 4 causes of hyperkalaemia   *2 marks*

1.

2.

3.

4.

Give 2 ECG changes associated with hyperkalaemia   *1 mark*

1.

2.

Urological

133

How would you treat life-threatening hyperkalaemia?   **3 marks**

1.

2.

3.

Friso's hyperkalaemia does not warrant urgent treatment. He undergoes nephrostomy to relieve his upper urinary tract obstruction and his ureteric stone is successfully fragmented by extracorporeal shockwave lithotripsy (ESWL). His urea and electrolyte data subsequently indicate recovery of his renal function.

Name 2 early complications following recovery from acute renal failure **2 marks**

1.

2.

Total: **20 marks**

Urological

ANSWERS
PAGES 303–308

CARDIOVASCULAR CASES:
ANSWERS

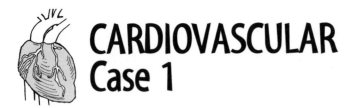

CARDIOVASCULAR
Case 1

Edwin, a 58-year-old KLM pilot, is brought into A&E by ambulance. He has a 45-minute history of central, crushing chest pain associated with nausea, dyspnoea and sweating. On cardiovascular system examination, his blood pressure is 154/96 mmHg, heart rate is 84 bpm and regular; the jugular venous pulse is 4 cm above the sternal angle, the apex beat is not displaced, heart sounds are normal and the chest is clear.

List 6 differential diagnoses   ***3 marks***

1. **Myocardial infarction.**

2. **Angina pectoris.**

3. **Pulmonary embolism.**

4. **Aortic dissection.**

5. **Gastro-oesophageal reflux disease.**

6. **Pericarditis.**

7. **Musculoskeletal chest pain.**

QUESTIONS
PAGES 1–4

137

The ECG is shown:

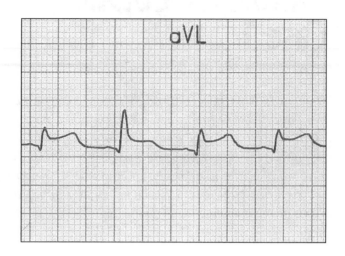

What is the abnormality? *1 mark*

1. ST-segment elevation.

This abnormality is seen in leads I, aVL and V5/V6.

What is the likely diagnosis? *2 marks*

1. Lateral wall (1 mark) myocardial infarction (1 mark).

What 2 other ECG changes may be expected to develop? *1 mark*

1. T wave inversion (within 24 hours).

2. Pathological Q waves (within days).

What 4 brief questions would you ask? **2 marks**

1. Any history of coronary heart disease (CHD)?

2. Any risk factors for CHD? (1 mark in total for specific risk factors)

3. Any existing drugs for CHD?

4. Any contraindications for thrombolysis?

What is your immediate management? **4 marks**

1. O$_2$: to ensure maximal oxygenation of myocardium.

2. Aspirin (300 mg chewed if not given already), or clopidogrel if aspirin is contraindicated: provides antiplatelet activity.

3. Sublingual glyceryl trinitrate (spray or tablets): to ensure maximal coronary artery vasodilatation.

4. Diamorphine iv (+ antiemetic): provides analgesia plus vasodilatation.

5. Thrombolysis: to achieve reperfusion of coronary arteries. Streptokinase is the agent most commonly used, though anterior myocardial infarctions (MIs) are thrombolysed with tissue plasminogen activator or tenecteplase.

6. Intravenous ß-blocker: reduces risk of sudden death.

Other than full blood count and urea and electrolytes, what 4 other investigations would you do? **4 marks**

1. Lipids: hyperlipidaemia is a risk factor for CHD.

2. Glucose: diabetes mellitus is a risk factor for CHD.

3. Cardiac enzymes or troponin T (12 hours after onset): to confirm MI.

4. Chest X-ray: to exclude pulmonary causes of chest pain; signs of heart failure.

The patient undergoes thrombolysis with streptokinase within 4 hours.

List 2 indications for thrombolysis **2 marks**

1. **ST-segment elevation > 2 mm in 2 contiguous chest leads.**

2. **ST-segment elevation > 1 mm in 2 limb leads.**

3. **New-onset left bundle branch block (LBBB). New LBBB is usually the result of a large anterior infarct.**

Name 3 <u>absolute</u> contraindications for thrombolysis **3 marks**

1. **Aortic dissection.**

2. **Recent stroke: stroke within the past 6 months or any previous haemorrhagic stroke.**

3. **Recent serious trauma, head injury or surgery (within 3 weeks).**

4. **Serious active bleeding (not menstrual).**

5. **Intracranial neoplasm.**

6. **Unconscious.**

Edwin is discharged 5 days later with no complications.

What advice, treatment and investigations would you recommend to reduce his risk of a similar episode? **3 marks**

1. **Echocardiogram: to assess any structural/functional heart defects.**

2. **Exercise ECG: any risk of exercise-induced ECG changes?**

3. **Coronary angiogram (depending on exercise test result): to assess extent of CHD.**

4. **Address any modifiable risk factors, eg smoking, hypertension, hypercholesterolaemia, diabetes mellitus. (½ mark in total for individual risk factors)**

5. Supervised cardiac rehabilitation.

6. Angiotensin converting enzyme inhibitor: minimises left ventricular impairment. Consider its use in all patients with MI, but certainly use it in cases of left ventricular failure or extensive myocardial damage.

7. Aspirin 75 mg daily: reduces risk of all vascular events (if contraindicated, consider clopidogrel).

8. Oral ß-blocker: reduces mortality in patients with MI.

9. Statin therapy: shown to improve prognosis regardless of baseline cholesterol concentration.

10. Omega-3.

Total: *25 marks*

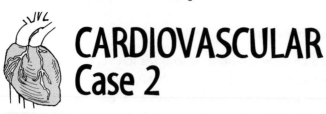

CARDIOVASCULAR
Case 2

Sarah, a 77-year-old retired dog breeder, presents to A&E with a 6-hour history of palpitations and feeling faint. On cardiovascular system examination her heart rate is 120 bpm, blood pressure is 130/90 mmHg; the jugular venous pulse is not raised and the apex beat not displaced; she has a systolic murmur, principally in the 5th intercostal space midclavicular line; the chest is clear.

Her ECG is shown below:

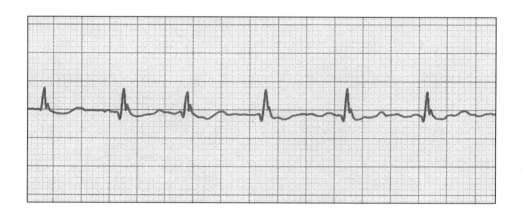

What does the ECG show? **1 mark**

1. Atrial fibrillation.

🔵 Absent P waves, irregular QRS complexes.

QUESTIONS
PAGES 5–7

List 4 causes of this rhythm   **2 marks**

1. Hypertension.

2. Ischaemic heart disease.

3. Cardiomyopathy.

4. Hyperthyroidism.

5. Mitral valve disease.

6. Pneumonia.

7. Alcohol excess.

8. Acute pulmonary embolism.

9. Lone atrial fibrillation.

What is the likely murmur?   **1 mark**

1. Mitral regurgitation.

Mitral regurgitation causes a pansystolic murmur that merges with the 2nd heart sound and is best heard over the mitral region – ie 5th intercostal space midclavicular line. Other causes of pansystolic murmurs are tricuspid regurgitation and ventricular septal defect.

What 6 other investigations would you do?   **6 marks**

1. Full blood count: any indication of infection.

2. Urea and electrolytes: any electrolyte imbalance, eg hypokalaemia, potentiates the toxicity of digoxin.

3. Thyroid function tests: to exclude hyperthyroidism.

continues . . .

4. Chest X-ray: to exclude heart failure, pneumonia.

5. Cardiac enzymes/troponin T: to exclude myocardial infarction.

6. Echocardiogram: to assess valvular disease, to assess structure of the heart.

7. Clotting screen/international normalised ratio (INR): in preparation for anticoagulation.

What 2 drugs may be used to slow down her ventricular rate?   *2 marks*

1. Digoxin.

2. ß-Blocker.

3. Calcium channel blocker.

⬤ Consider amiodarone in resistant cases.

Sarah's abnormal rhythm fails to resolve on rate reduction.

What 2 methods may be used to attempt cardioversion?   *2 marks*

1. Antiarrhythmic drugs, eg amiodarone (class 3 antiarrhythmic drug that acts by inhibiting repolarisation) or flecainide. Side-effects of amiodarone include hyper- and hypothyroidism, deranged liver function tests and pulmonary fibrosis.

2. DC cardioversion: may be performed as an emergency if the patient is haemodynamically compromised. If the atrial fibrillation is of recent onset (< 48 hours) and the heart is normal on echocardiography, there is no need to anticoagulate before cardioversion; otherwise, anticoagulate 4 weeks before and 4–6 weeks after cardioversion.

What 3 signs/symptoms would suggest that Sarah is haemodynamically compromised?   *3 marks*

1. Hypotension (systolic blood pressure < 90 mmHg).

2. Heart failure (eg basal crackles); jugular venous pulse raised.

3. Chest pain.

4. Tachypnoea.

5. Impaired consciousness.

6. Heart rate uncontrolled.

In the event of compromise, what are the first 2 things you should do?   **2 marks**

1. Give O_2.

2. Summon expert help.

Name 3 complications if her abnormal rhythm is not appropriately treated?

3 marks

1. Cerebrovascular accident (stroke).

2. Heart failure.

3. Syncope.

4. Angina.

What drug is used to prevent embolic events, how is it monitored and what is the target range?   **3 marks**

1. Warfarin.

2. INR (normal range is 0.9–1.2). It is calculated by comparing the prothrombin time of the patient against a standard value.

3. 2–3.

Total: **25 marks**

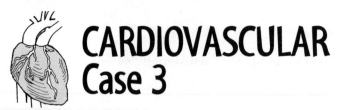

CARDIOVASCULAR
Case 3

Durk, a 54-year-old butcher, has attended his GP for his third blood pressure measurement; his three readings are 167/96, 162/104 and 174/104 mmHg. With regards to his medical history, he is asthmatic and has a body mass index of 28 kg/m².

Define the systolic/diastolic ranges for mild (phase 1), moderate (phase 2) and severe (phase 3) hypertension   **3 marks**

1. Mild: **140–159/90–99 mmHg.**

2. Moderate: **160–199/100–109 mmHg.**

3. Severe: **≥ 200/110 mmHg.**

🛈 Treat moderate to severe hypertension; treat mild hypertension if there is target-organ damage, cardiovascular disease (CVD), diabetes mellitus (DM) or 10-year coronary heart disease risk ≥ 15% (calculated on the basis of sex, smoking status, DM and total cholesterol : high-density lipoprotein ratio).

List 3 causes of secondary hypertension   **3 marks**

1. Renal disease, eg renal artery stenosis, glomerulonephritis.

2. Endocrine disorders: Conn's syndrome (hyperaldosteronism), Cushing's syndrome (corticosteroid excess), phaeochromocytoma (excess noradrenaline and adrenaline), acromegaly (growth hormone excess).

3. Drugs: combined oral contraceptive, corticosteroids, alcohol.

4. Aortic coarctation.

5. Pregnancy.

QUESTIONS
PAGES 8–11

What 3 questions would you ask? **3 marks**

1. Any family history of hypertension?

2. Any personal/family history of renal disease, eg polycystic kidneys?

3. Any risk factors for cardiovascular disease, eg smoking, DM?

4. Any medications that may cause secondary hypertension?

5. Any contraindications for treatment? (For example, ß-blockers are contraindicated in asthma, and thiazides are contraindicated in the presence of severely impaired renal function, gout and DM.)

What 6 initial investigations would you do? **3 marks**

1. Full blood count: normocytic anaemia may be associated with chronic renal failure (which may be a result of, or a cause of, hypertension).

2. Urea and electrolytes (U&Es): exclude impaired renal function; hypokalaemia may indicate Conn's syndrome.

3. Fasting lipids: hypercholesterolaemia is an independent risk factor for CVD.

4. Fasting glucose: DM is an independent risk factor for CVD.

5. Urine dipstick for protein and blood: may indicate renal disease (if positive, send for microscopy and request renal ultrasound scan).

6. ECG: may indicate previous myocardial infarction; left ventricular hypertrophy (LVH) (eg left axis deviation, tall R waves in V5/6) indicates end-organ damage (request chest X-ray if signs of heart disease).

7. Chest X-ray (normal, cardiomegaly, pulmonary oedema, coarctation).

Durk's ECG is shown:

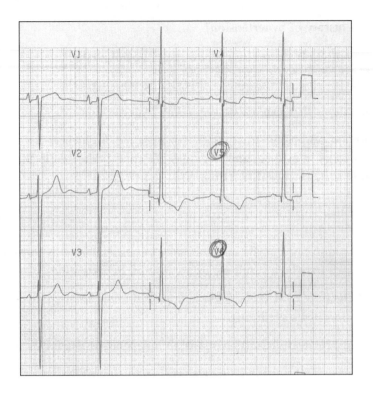

What does his ECG show?   *1 mark*

1. The ECG shows LVH.

ⓘ LVH causes tall R waves in V5/V6 and deep S waves in V1/V2 (consider
LVH if the R wave in V5/V6 is > 25 mm or the combined R wave in V6
and S wave in V1 are > 35 mm). May also get T wave inversion in the
lateral leads (ie I, VL, V5/V6) and left axis deviation (ie positive in I,
negative in II and III).

Would this ECG influence your treatment in someone with hypertension and, if
so, why?   *1 mark*

**1. LVH indicates hypertensive end-organ damage and is an indication for
antihypertensive treatment in a patient with increased blood pressure.**

ⓘ End-organ damage is an indication for antihypertensive treatment, even in patients with mild hypertension.

What 3 lifestyle changes would you recommend? **3 marks**

1. Lose weight – aim for body mass index 20–25 kg/m².

2. Stop smoking.

3. Encourage regular exercise.

4. Reduce salt consumption.

5. Reduce alcohol consumption to < 21 units/week.

Name 2 appropriate antihypertensive drugs that may be prescribed to reduce Durk's blood pressure **2 marks**

1. Low-dose thiazide, eg 2.5 mg bendrofluazide.

2. Angiotensin converting enzyme inhibitor (ACEI), eg ramipril.

3. Calcium channel blocker, eg amlodipine.

ⓘ ß-Blockers are contraindicated (potentially fatal) in Durk's case, as he is asthmatic – fail the <u>complete</u> question if prescribed.

Durk is prescribed an ACEI by his GP.

What 2 abnormalities on U&E may an ACEI cause? **1 mark**

1. Hyperkalaemia: as a result of inhibition of aldosterone-mediated excretion of K⁺.

2. Increased urea and creatinine: may cause impaired renal function as a result of reduced renal perfusion in patients with renovascular disease; use with caution if generalised atherosclerosis or peripheral vascular disease present.

ⓘ When an ACEI is being prescribed, U&Es must be monitored at baseline, 1–2 weeks after initiation of treatment, after every increase in dose and at annual review.

List 3 circumstances in which you would consider referring a hypertensive patient for specialist care **3 marks**

1. Suspicion of secondary hypertension.

2. Young, eg < 35 years.

3. Impaired renal function.

4. Proteinuria or haematuria, or both.

5. Hypokalaemia (in the absence of diuretics).

6. Refractory hypertension to multiple combined antihypertensive medications (exclude poor compliance).

7. Accelerated phased (malignant) hypertension, ie blood pressure > 200/140 mmHg + bilateral retinal haemorrhages and cotton wool spots (papilloedema may or may not be present).

Name 4 complications if Durk's hypertension is not treated **2 marks**

1. Stroke: hypertensive individuals have a 6-fold greater risk of stroke than normotensive people.

2. CVD: hypertensive individuals have a 3-fold greater risk of CVD than normotensive people.

3. Heart failure.

4. Peripheral vascular disease.

5. Chronic renal failure: hypertensive nephropathy.

6. Impaired vision: hypertensive retinopathy.

Total: **25 marks**

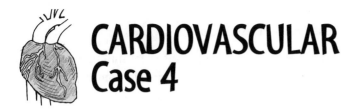

CARDIOVASCULAR
Case 4

*Tim, a 60-year-old Professor of Endocrinology, visits his GP
complaining of recent episodes of central chest tightness at the end
of his golf rounds. These settle on rest and last no longer than
10–15 minutes. There is nothing of note in his past medical history.
Cardiovascular examination is normal.*

List 5 risk factors you would enquire about in the history   *5 marks*

**The probable diagnosis is angina pectoris, the main cause of which is coronary
heart disease (CHD).**

1. Smoking.

2. High-fat, low-fruit and low-vegetable diet.

3. Sedentary lifestyle.

4. Diabetes mellitus.

5. Hypertension.

6. Hyperlipidaemia.

7. Family history of CHD.

What 4 initial blood tests would you do and why?   *4 marks*

1. Full blood count: to exclude anaemia as a cause of his angina.

2. Thyroid function tests: to exclude hyperthyroidism as a cause of his angina.

3. Glucose: diabetes mellitus is a risk factor for CHD.

? QUESTIONS
PAGES 12–15

4. Fasting lipids: hyperlipidaemia is a risk factor for CHD.

5. Urea and electrolytes (U&Es): to exclude impaired renal function, which is a relative contraindication for ACEI and low-dose thiazide therapy; if the patient is hypertensive, impaired renal function may be a cause of, or a result of, high blood pressure.

6. Liver function tests (LFTs): statins are contraindicated in active liver disease.

All these blood tests prove normal, except a fasting total cholesterol (TC) of 7.2 mmol/l.

What is the recommended upper limit for fasting TC in the secondary prevention of CHD?   *1 mark*

1. 5 mmol/l.

🛈 Patients with existing CHD should ideally have a fasting TC ≤ 5 mmol/l (or a 30% reduction, whichever is greatest) (and a low-density cholesterol ≤ 3 mmol/l). In patients without CHD – ie in primary prevention – patients with a 10-year CHD risk greater than 15% (tables to calculate this risk are presented in the back of the *British National Formulary*) should also have TC ≤ 5 mmol/l.

Tim is prescribed a statin by his GP.

What blood test must you request before prescribing a statin and what advice must you give patients receiving statin therapy?   *2 marks*

1. LFTs.

🛈 Statins are potentially hepatotoxic and are contraindicated in liver impairment. LFTs should be carried out at baseline and at regular intervals thereafter; treatment should be discontinued if aspartate aminotransferase/alanine aminotransferase increases to 3x the upper limit of normal (normal range is 3–35 iu/l).

2. Patients should report any unexplained muscle pain.

ⓘ Rarely, statins cause myopathy (diagnosed by increased creatinine kinase) causing muscle pain, weakness and tenderness.

Tim's resting ECG is normal. His GP arranges an outpatient appointment for him to undergo an exercise ECG to diagnose angina.

Indicate whether each of the following exercise ECGs represents a negative or positive exercise test **3 marks**

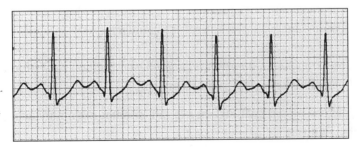

1.

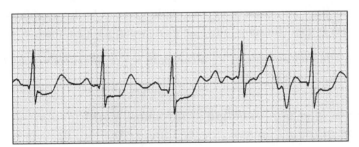

2.

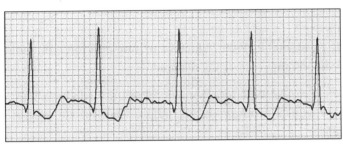

3.

1. ECG 1: **downsloping ST-segment depression is a positive exercise test.**

3. ECG 3: **planar ST-segment depression is a positive exercise test.**

2. ECG 2: **upsloping ST-segment depression is a negative exercise test.**

🛈 Horizontal or downsloping ST-segment depression (assessed at the J point, which is two small squares after the S wave) indicates myocardial ischaemia.

Tim's exercise ECG is positive and a diagnosis of stable angina is made. The cardiologist prescribes aspirin 75 mg od, addresses his modifiable risk factors and places him on the waiting list for coronary angiography.

List 3 drugs that may be prescribed to control angina **3 marks**

1. **ß-Blockers, eg atenolol: these reduce heart rate and force of contraction, thereby reducing myocardial O$_2$ demand.**

2. **Nitrates: these are vasodilators. For symptoms, use sublingual glyceryl trinitrate spray; as a prophylaxis, give regular oral nitrate, eg isosorbide mononitrate.**

3. **Calcium channel antagonists, eg amlodipine: act as both vasodilators and negative inotropes (thereby reducing myocardial O$_2$ demand).**

4. **Potassium channel activators, eg nicorandil: hyperpolarise the membrane, thereby reducing heart rate.**

Six months later, Tim undergoes angiography, which shows severe occlusion of the left anterior descending (LAD) artery.

What 2 procedures are available to treat the stenosed LAD? **2 marks**

1. **Percutaneous transluminal coronary angioplasty: balloon dilatation of the stenosed vessel, usually with stent insertion.**

2. **Coronary artery bypass grafting: eg use left internal mammary artery to bypass the stenosis.**

Total: **20 marks**

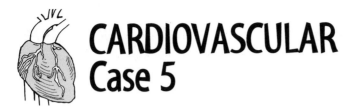

CARDIOVASCULAR
Case 5

Clint, a 72-year-old retired army major, is referred by his GP to the cardiac outpatient department complaining of a 3-month history of progressive breathlessness. He is now breathless even when doing simple tasks around the home, such as ironing. With regards to his past medical history, he is receiving treatment for hypertension and rheumatoid arthritis.

List 4 non-cardiac causes of gradually progressive dyspnoea **2 marks**

1. Chronic obstructive pulmonary disease.

2. Fibrotic lung disease, eg occupational lung disease, granulomatous disease (eg sarcoidosis), connective tissue disease (eg rheumatoid arthritis).

3. Lung cancer.

4. Pleural effusion.

5. Anaemia.

6. Multiple pulmonary emboli.

From the history above, classify his heart failure according to the New York Health Association criteria **1 mark**

1. Grade III heart failure, ie dyspnoea on minimal exertion.

New York Heart Association heart failure classification

Grade	Extent of breathlessness
I	No undue breathlessness
II	Breathlessness on moderate exertion
III	**Dyspnoea on minimal exertion**
IV	Dyspnoea at rest; all activity causes discomfort

QUESTIONS
PAGES 16–19

List 4 symptoms suggestive of left ventricular failure (LVF)   **2 marks**

1. Fatigue.

2. Exertional dyspnoea.

3. Orthopnoea: enquire about the number of pillows slept on at night.

4. Paroxysmal nocturnal dyspnoea: patient complains of waking up with sensation of drowning.

5. Nocturnal cough (may bring up pink froth).

6. 'Cardiac' wheeze.

ⓘ Symptoms of right ventricular failure (RVF) include fatigue, peripheral oedema, anorexia and nausea (due to bowel oedema), abdominal distension (due to ascites), right upper quadrant pain (caused by liver congestion), wasting (often with fluid-derived weight gain).

What hormone is significantly increased in heart failure?   **1 mark**

1. B-Type (or brain) natriuretic peptide (BNP).

ⓘ BNP is secreted by the ventricular myocardium in response to distension and acts to reduce circulating volume by inhibiting renin, antidiuretic hormone and aldosterone secretion (actions similar to those of atrial natriuretic peptide). Concentrations are significantly increased in heart failure and BNP is now (where available) being used as a screening test for heart failure.

What key investigation would you do to confirm heart failure?   **1 mark**

1. Echocardiogram: this is the key investigation in heart failure. It will confirm the diagnosis and its severity, and may indicate the cause, eg aortic stenosis.

ⓘ Other investigations include: full blood count (exclude anaemia), urea and electrolytes (hypoalbuminaemia and renal failure cause fluid retention; preparation for angiotensin converting enzyme inhibitor (ACEI)/diuretic therapy), thyroid function tests (exclude hyper-/hypothyroidism), liver function tests (hepatic congestion), glucose and lipids (risk factors for ischaemic heart disease, the main cause of heart failure), ECG (may show the cause, eg myocardial infarction), chest X-ray. Cardiac enzymes/troponin T (in an acute setting).

Clint is diagnosed with left ventricular failure.

Clint's posteroanterior chest X-ray is shown:

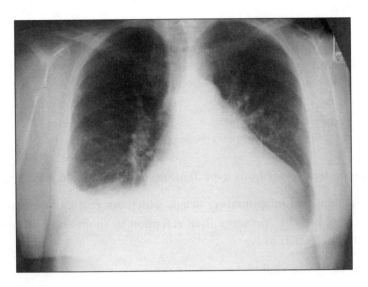

List 4 features seen on Clint's posteroanterior chest X-ray   *2 marks*

1. **Cardiomegaly: > 50% of cardiac : thoracic ratio (not possible to assess on anteroposterior film).**

2. **Fluid in horizontal fissure: seen as horizontal white line in right lung field.**

3. **Pleural effusions: blunting of costophrenic angles.**

4. **Upper lobe diversion: prominent vascular markings in upper lung fields.**

5. **Interstitial oedema: seen as small faint horizontal white lines at peripheries of lung fields (Kerley's B lines).**

🔵 There is no evidence of frank pulmonary oedema.

List 4 causes of LVF   *2 marks*

1. **Ischaemic heart disease.**

2. **Myocardial infarction.**

3. **Hypertension.**

4. **Left-sided valve disease, eg aortic stenosis, severe mitral regurgitation, aortic regurgitation.**

5. **Cardiomyopathies, eg dilated cardiomyopathy.**

🛈 The main causes of RVF are secondary to LVF, cor pulmonale, pulmonary embolism, right-sided valve disease, left-to-right shunts, eg ventricular septal defect.

What 3 medications may be exacerbating Clint's LVF?   *3 marks*

Clint is being treated for both hypertension and rheumatoid arthritis.

1. **Non-steroidal anti-inflammatory drugs, which are first-line therapy for rheumatoid arthritis, promote fluid retention by inhibiting prostaglandin-mediated excretion of Na^+.**

2. **ß-Blockers, eg atenolol.**

3. **Calcium channel blockers, eg verapamil.**

🛈 Both ß-blockers and calcium channel blockers are commonly used antihypertensive drugs which are negative inotropes and will further suppress left ventricular function. In stable heart failure, ß-blockers are introduced in low dose, with slow, stepwise titration to improve long-term prognosis.

Clint is initially prescribed an angiotensin converting enzyme inhibitor (ACEI) and frusemide.

List 3 electrolyte abnormalities caused by frusemide   *3 marks*

Frusemide is a loop diuretic that acts by inhibiting the $Na^+/K^+/2Cl^-$ pump in the loop of Henlé. It may cause:

1. **Hyponatraemia.**

2. **Hypocalcaemia (unlike thiazides, which are calcium-sparing diuretics).**

3. **Hypokalaemia (if this is problematic, consider giving frusemide in combination with a potassium-sparing diuretic, though ACEIs cause hyperkalaemia, so this is not usually necessary).**

4. **Hypomagnesaemia.**

5. **Hyperuricaemia.**

Although his frusemide and ACEI therapy is optimised, Clint remains symptomatic, so his cardiologist adds spironolactone and digoxin to his medication.

What electrolyte abnormality potentiates digoxin toxicity?   *1 mark*

1. Hypokalaemia potentiates digoxin toxicity.

🔅 Digoxin inhibits the Na^+/K^+ pump, resulting in increased intracellular Ca^{2+} (in exchange for Na^+). This increases the force of myocardial contraction. It also stimulates parasympathetic innervation, reducing the heart rate. Digoxin has a very narrow therapeutic range (1.3–2.6 nmol/l). Toxicity causes anorexia, nausea, visual disturbance and arrhythmias, eg ventricular tachycardia. This is treated by stopping the drug, correcting any hypokalaemia and treating any arrhythmia (in life-threatening toxicity, anti-digoxin specific antibody fragments may be used).

What 2 electrolyte abnormalites does digoxin toxicity cause?   *1 mark*

1. Hyperkalaemia.

2. Hyponatraemia.

🔅 This the result of inhibition of the Na^+/K^+ pump at the cellular level, preventing cellular uptake of K^+ in exchange for Na^+.

Total: **20 marks**

ENDOCRINOLOGY CASES:
ANSWERS

ENDOCRINOLOGY
Case 1

Imke, a 38-year-old child psychologist, is referred by her GP to the endocrinologists; she has symptoms of hyperthyroidism.

Name 6 symptoms Imke may be complaining of　　　　　　　　　**3 marks**

1. Weight loss, increased appetite.

2. Diarrhoea.

3. Heat intolerance.

4. Sweating.

5. Fatigue.

6. Palpitations, dyspnoea, angina.

7. Irritability, nervousness, restlessness, insomnia.

8. Oligomenorrhoea, infertility.

9. Eye complaints, eg diplopia, reduced visual acuity.

On examination she is in fast atrial fibrillation, and has a diffuse goitre and bulging eyes.

List 4 signs specific to Graves' disease　　　　　　　　　　　　**2 marks**

Signs of thyroid disease include tachycardia, atrial fibrillation, warm vasodilated peripheries, fine tremor, eyelid lag and goitre (either diffuse or nodular). Graves' disease is associated with additional signs:

QUESTIONS
PAGES 23–26

1. **Exophthalmus, ie protruding eyes.**

2. **Ophthalmoplegia, ie paralysis of extraocular muscles causing strabismus: due to muscle swelling and fibrosis.**

3. **Conjunctival oedema.**

4. **Periorbital oedema.**

5. **Pretibial myxoedema, ie oedematous swelling of shins.**

6. **Thyroid acropathy, ie clubbing.**

7. **Thyroid bruit.**

What is the underlying cause of Graves' disease?   *2 marks*

1. **Thyroid-stimulating hormone (TSH) receptor antibodies binding to the TSH receptor, stimulating production of thyroid hormones.**

❶ Graves' disease is the most common cause of hyperthyroidism, causing relapsing and remitting hyperthyroidism that often eventually progresses to hypothyroidism. It is associated with other autoimmune conditions such as pernicious anaemia, type 1 diabetes and myasthenia gravis.

❶ Other causes of hyperthyroidism include toxic adenoma (Plummer's disease), toxic multinodular goitre, thyroiditis (transient hyperthyroidism as a result of acute inflammation of gland), thyroid cancer and drugs (eg excess thyroxine, amiodarone).

Bloods are taken for thyroid function tests and thyroid-stimulating hormone (TSH) receptor antibodies, confirming the diagnosis of Graves' disease. Her thyroid function test results are shown below.

Indicate (↑, ↓ or →) at '?' the expected changes   *3 marks*

	Normal range	Expected change
TSH	0.5–5.7 munit/l	↓
T4	70–140 nmol/l	↑
T3	1.2–3.0 nmol/l	↑

(TSH = thyroid-stimulating hormone, T3 = tri-iodothyronine, T4 = thyroxine)

🛈 Other investigations in hyperthyroidism may include: erythrocyte sedimentation rate (increased in thyroiditis), a thyroid scan to identify any solitary or multinodular goitre, fine-needle aspiration of any nodules for cytology, and radiolabelled iodine scan to assess thyroid uptake, ie hot or cold nodules (increased risk of cancer in cold nodules).

Imke is anticoagulated; her symptoms are treated with ß-blockers, and her hyperthyroidism by a 'block and replace' regimen with carbimazole and thyroxine.

Give 2 short-term and 2 long-term complications if her hyperthyroidism is untreated   **4 marks**

Short-term complications:

1. Stroke: the risk of embolic stroke is high in atrial fibrillation associated with hyperthyroidism, and anticoagulation is mandatory.

2. Angina.

3. Myocardial infarction.

4. Thyrotoxic storm.

Long-term complications:

1. Osteoporosis.

2. Heart failure due to increased cardiac output.

🛈 Thyroid crisis (thyrotoxic storm) is the result of a rapid deterioration of hyperthyroidism causing fast atrial fibrillation, hyperthermia, confusion and coma. It may be triggered by myocardial infarction, trauma, infection or thyroid surgery (prevented by ensuring the patient is euthyroid before surgery).

🛈 The eye problems of Graves' disease are typically independent of the thyroid status and are therefore not prevented by treating the hyperthyroidism. Treatment may involve taping eyelids closed at night, use of lubricating eye-drops, lateral tarsorrhaphy (to protect the cornea), high-dose corticosteroids and surgical decompression of the orbit.

Give 4 indications for thyroidectomy in Imke   *2 marks*

1. Patient choice, eg for cosmetic reasons.

2. Pressure symptoms from a large goitre, eg dyspnoea, dysphagia.

3. Intolerable side-effects of drugs; eg carbimazole may cause agranulocytosis (propylthiouracil is an alternative treatment, but may also cause suppression of the bone marrow).

4. Poor compliance with drug treatment.

5. Relapse of hyperthyroidism after withdrawal of medication (patients are usually treated for 12–18 months).

ⓘ In nodular goitre, a further indication for surgery is risk of thyroid cancer on the basis of fine-needle aspiration of any nodule or presence of cold nodules on radiolabelled iodine uptake scan.

Give 4 complications of surgery   *2 marks*

1. Early postoperative bleeding causing dyspnoea as a result of pressure effects from haematoma.

2. Hypothyroidism.

3. Recurrent hyperthyroidism.

4. Hypoparathyroidism causing hypocalcaemia (due to damage to adjacent parathyroid glands).

5. Hoarseness caused by damage to the recurrent laryngeal nerve.

On cessation of the 'block and replace' regimen, Imke remains hyperthyroid. She is subsequently treated with radioactive iodine, which initially renders her euthyroid, though eventually leaves her hypothyroid.

List 4 other causes of hypothyroidism   *2 marks*

1. **Autoimmune hypothyroidism, eg Hashimoto's thyroiditis, atrophic hypothyroidism.**

2. **Iodine deficiency.**

3. **Thyroidectomy.**

4. **Drugs, eg antithyroid drugs, amiodarone.**

5. **Congenital: screened for by the Guthrie test at postnatal day 7 (detects increased TSH in heel-prick sample).**

Total: *20 marks*

ENDOCRINOLOGY
Case 2

Lysbet, aged 12 years, is seen by her GP after a 3-day history of polyuria, polydipsia, lethargy and recent weight loss, and now complaining of abdominal pain and occasional vomiting. Urine dipstick showed glycosuria and ketonuria and she was admitted to the children's ward. On examination, her Glasgow Coma Scale score is 15/15, her heart rate is 120 bpm; her abdomen is tender throughout, she is hyperventilating and she appears moderately dehydrated.

How is diabetic ketoacidosis (DKA) diagnosed biochemically?   *3 marks*

1. Hyperglycaemia: blood glucose > 11 mmol/l.

2. Ketonuria.

3. Acidosis: blood pH < 7.25.

ℹ️ Type 1 diabetes typically presents with the classical symptoms of polyuria, polydipsia, weight loss and lethargy, but it may also present with DKA. This is due to hyperglycaemia secondary to insulin deficiency, which causes osmotic diuresis resulting in dehydration; deficiency of intracellular glucose switches energy production to lipolysis, which forms ketone bodies (detected as ketonuria), causing metabolic acidosis (which is associated with abdominal pain and vomiting, further exacerbating fluid and electrolyte balance). A diagnosis of DKA requires all 3 biochemical changes to be present.

Lysbet is diagnosed with DKA. Her venous blood gases are shown below.

QUESTIONS
PAGES 27–30

Indicate (↑, ↓ or →) at '?' the expected changes   *3 marks*

	Normal range	Lysbet's gases	Explanation
pH	7.35–7.45	↓	Acidosis due to ketonaemia
pO_2	10–12 kPa	11	Depending on whether patient is shocked, hypoxia may or may not be present
pCO_2	4.7–6 kPa	↓	Hypocapnia due to respiratory compensation causing hyperventilation
HCO_3^-	22–28 mmol/l	↓	Bicarbonate-depleted attempting to buffer metabolic acidosis
BE	± 2 mmol/l	-5	Base deficit due to HCO_3^- depletion

(BE = base excess)

Lysbet is successfully treated with iv 0.9% saline and iv insulin.

List 3 complications of this treatment   *3 marks*

1. Hypokalaemia: due to insulin driving potassium into cells. This is minimised by addition of KCl to iv fluids. This may cause arrhythmias.

2. Hypoglycaemia: due to excessive insulin therapy. This may cause hypoglycaemic coma.

3. Hypernatraemia: due to excessive iv saline. This is minimised by changing to 0.45% saline + 5% dextrose.

4. Fluid overload: may cause pulmonary and/or cerebral oedema.

List 2 causes of DKA in a child known to have type 1 diabetes   *2 marks*

1. Interruption of insulin therapy, eg non-compliance.

2. Infection.

3. Surgery.

🛈 Examples 2 and 3 above can cause DKA as a result of stress, increasing the insulin demand. All patients receive illness rules to minimise the risk of DKA (see below).

Once Lysbet's condition has stabilised, she and her parents are seen by the diabetes nurse, who starts her on insulin therapy and educates them on the management of diabetes mellitus.

List 4 'illness rules' you would give Lysbet   **2 marks**

1. Obtain early treatment for infections.

2. Always take your insulin therapy.

3. Self-monitor more often during illnesses and adjust therapy accordingly (or seek advice if hyperglycaemic).

4. If unable to eat (eg anorexia, nauseous), take sweet fluids in place of meals.

5. Take plenty of sugar-free fluids frequently, to prevent dehydration.

🛈 Infections, due to the increased stress on the body, increase insulin demand and may lead to a loss of glycaemic control, potentially causing DKA. This may be exacerbated by the common misconception that if the patient is not eating properly there is no need for them to take their insulin.

List 4 warning signs of hypoglycaemia   **2 marks**

Autonomic:

1. Sweating, palpitations, shaking, hunger.

Neurological:

2. Confusion, drowsiness, inco-ordination, odd behaviour, slurred speech.

🛈 The brain depends on a constant supply of glucose to maintain function; a concentration < 3.5 mmol/l impairs neurological function. This activates the sympathetic nervous system, which opposes the actions of insulin and warns the patient. Risk is increased by missed meals and unusual exertion. All patients with type 1 diabetes should carry rapidly absorbed carbohydrate and a warning card.

What 2 co-existing conditions should you screen for in Lysbet? **2 marks**

1. Hyper- and hypothyroidism: excluded by thyroid function tests.

2. Coeliac disease: excluded by anti-gliadin antibody screen.

🛈 Type 1 diabetes, an autoimmune disease, is associated with thyroid and coeliac disease, the presence of which complicates good glycaemic control. These should be screened for at diagnosis and regular intervals throughout life.

How is long-term glycaemic control assessed and what value indicates good control? **2 marks**

1. Glycaemic control over the previous 8 weeks, ie the half-life of a red blood cell, is assessed by glycated haemoglobin (HbA1c).

2. HbA1c < 7% reflects good control.

Interpretation	HbA1c (%)
Hypoglycaemic risk	< 4.1
Normal range (difficult to achieve without frequent hypoglycaemia)	4.1–6.1
Good control	6.2–7
Increasing risk	> 7

List 4 challenges facing Lysbet and her family **4 marks**

🛈 There are no 'correct' answers to this question. However, it has been included to highlight the fact that diabetes mellitus is a self-managed disease and if the child is unwilling or unable to self-manage their own diabetes the outcome is poor. The greatest barrier to good self-management in children (and adults) are the challenges posed by diabetes mellitus, which may be specific to diabetes mellitus or chronic diseases in general. A few examples are shown (be strict when awarding marks!):

1. **Managing medical treatment: eg regular blood tests and self-injecting may stigmatise the child.**

2. **Fear regarding the future: complications of diabetes mellitus, both short-term, eg regular blood tests, and long-term, eg blindness.**

3. **The need for regular meals takes away the child's (and family's) spontaneity.**

4. **Family relations: places a large strain on the family, eg siblings may feel left out.**

Lysbet is screened annually to monitor the long-term complications of diabetes mellitus.

List 2 annual screening tests Lysbet should undergo   *2 marks*

1. **Blood pressure monitoring: all children should be screened for hypertension from 12 years of age. Increased blood pressure increases the risk of macro- and microvascular complications of diabetes mellitus; the target is 130/80 mmHg. Angiotensin converting enzyme inhibitors are the first-line treatment as they also reduce the risk of nephropathy.**

2. **Urine dipstick for microalbuminuria or albumin : creatinine (A : C) ratio in first-pass urine sample. If the dipstick test is positive (or A : C increased to > 2.5), perform 24-hour urine collection to quantify albumin excretion. Microalbuminuria (ie urinary albumin 30–300 mg/d) indicates an increased risk of diabetic nephropathy (defined as albuminuria > 300 mg/d) and the need for tighter glycaemic control.**

3. **Retinal screening for diabetic retinopathy characterised by hard exudates, dot-and-blot haemorrhages, cotton wool spots and formation of new vessels on retina.**

🛈 Children with diabetes mellitus should undergo annual screening from the age of 12 years for retinopathy, hypertension and microalbuminaemia. There is no evidence that screening for hyperlipidaemia is of benefit.

Total: *25 marks*

GASTROINTESTINAL CASES: ANSWERS

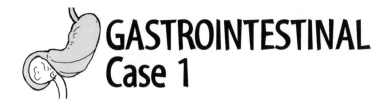

GASTROINTESTINAL
Case 1

George, a 46-year-old known alcoholic, presents to A&E with a 1-hour history of haematemesis, including a severe episode in the ambulance. On examination, his blood pressure is 86/44 mmHg, he is cold peripherally and his pulse is 110 bpm.

What is your immediate management?   **1 mark**

ABC, as the patient is shocked: heart rate > systolic blood pressure is a good working definition.

1. **Airways: protect airways by managing in the recovery position.**

2. **Breathing: give high-flow O$_2$.**

3. **Circulation: obtain iv access with 2 large-bore cannulae and resuscitate with iv saline/colloid/crystalloid while waiting for blood to be cross-matched (in emergencies can give group O Rhesus-negative blood).**

Which 2 colleagues should you call?   **1 mark**

1. **Call senior.**

2. **Warn surgeon on call of all serious bleeds.**

All patients should undergo an endoscopy within 24 hours of admission (within 4 hours if suspected variceal haemorrhage) for diagnosis, with or without surgical treatment. If there is severe or continuous bleeding, pass a Sengstaken-Blakemore tube to compress oesophageal varices (this should be attempted by your senior).

List 6 causes of haematemesis   **3 marks**

1. **Peptic ulcer disease.**

continues . . .

QUESTIONS
PAGES 33–36

2. Oesophageal varices.

3. Mallory-Weiss (oesophageal) tear: due to excessive vomiting.

4. Oesophagitis.

5. Gastritis.

6. Upper gastrointestinal (GI) malignancy, eg gastric cancer.

What 3 brief questions would you ask?   *3 marks*

1. **Any previous episodes of haematemesis and/or melaena (both indicate upper GI bleeds)? Include cause, severity and treatment.**

2. **Any known causes of upper GI bleeds, eg peptic ulcer disease, chronic liver disease?**

3. **Any dyspeptic symptoms, eg epigastric pain, gastro-oesophageal reflux disease?**

4. **Alcohol consumption, iv drug use: alcohol, hepatitis B virus (HBV) and hepatitis C virus (HCV) (from iv drug use) are the main causes of cirrhosis.**

5. **Medication history, eg non-steroidal anti-inflammatory drugs.**

What 4 blood tests would you request?   *2 marks*

1. **Full blood count (FBC): anaemia (haemoglobin may not decrease until circulating volume is restored), thrombocytopenia (increased risk of bleeding).**

2. **Urea and electrolytes (U&Es): any electrolyte abnormalities.**

3. **Clotting screen: any bleeding disorder, eg increased international normalised ratio (INR).**

4. **Liver function tests (LFTs): suspect varices if chronic liver disease; liver disease causes increased INR as a result of decreased clotting factor synthesis, decreased absorption of vitamin K (a fat-soluble vitamin requiring bile for absorption).**

5. **Cross match 4–6 units of blood.**

🛈 In the presence of a bleeding disorder, consult haematologist for advice on vitamin K injection, fresh frozen plasma and platelet transfusion.

George's history of chronic alcohol abuse and deranged liver function tests suggested a bleeding oesophageal varice as the cause of his haematemesis. As a result, he underwent emergency endoscopy, confirming a variceal haemorrhage that was successfully treated by variceal banding.

In patients with oesophageal varices, what drug is used as a prophylaxis against variceal haemorrhage? **1 mark**

1. ß-Blockers, eg propranolol: used to reduce portal hypertension.

🛈 Oesophageal varices are a result of portal hypertension (the most common cause in the UK is cirrhosis, the main cause of which is alcohol and chronic HCV/HBV infection).

Once his condition is stabilised, George is transferred to the wards for observation.

List 4 signs of a re-bleed while on the ward **2 marks**

1. Increasing heart rate.

2. Decreasing blood pressure.

3. Decreasing hourly urine output: patients should be catheterised so urinary output can be monitored; aim for output > 30 ml/h.

4. Haematemesis.

5. Melaena, or fresh p.r. bleeding.

What 2 blood tests may indicate that he has re-bled? **1 mark**

1. FBC: decreased haemoglobin.

2. U&Es: increased urea (with normal creatinine) – an upper GI bleed is equivalent to a large protein meal.

What 4 questions make up the CAGE questionnaire? **2 marks**

1. C: **have you ever felt that you should <u>c</u>ut down on your drinking?**

2. A: **have you ever been <u>a</u>nnoyed by people criticizing your drinking?**

3. G: **have you ever felt <u>g</u>uilty about your drinking?**

4. E: **do you need an <u>e</u>ye-opener (ie drink) to start the day?**

ⓘ The CAGE questionnaire is a quick screening tool for alcohol misuse. If ≥ 2 are positive, take a more detailed alcohol history.

List 2 blood tests to screen for alcohol misuse **1 mark**

1. **FBC: macrocytosis (ie mean corpuscular volume > 96 fl) with or without anaemia. Caused by a direct toxic effect of alcohol on the bone marrow, with or without vitamin B12/folate deficiency.**

2. **LFTs: increased γ-glutamyl transpeptidase.**

Name 6 other complications of alcohol misuse **3 marks**

Alcohol misuse causes numerous physical and psychosocial complications:

1. **Cardiovascular system: hypertension, heart failure (wet beriberi), cardiomyopathy, arrhythmias, anaemia.**

2. **Liver: hepatitis, cirrhosis.**

3. **GI: oesophageal cancer, peptic ulcer disease, pancreatitis.**

4. **Musculoskeletal: myopathy.**

5. **Nervous system: polyneuropathy, subacute combined degeneration, Wernicke-Korsakoff's syndrome, epilepsy, cerebellar degeneration, head injury (from falls).**

6. **Obstetric: fetal alcohol syndrome.**

7. **Social: accidents, violence, relationship and employment problems.**

8. **Psychiatric: depression, anxiety, suicide.**

Total: **20 marks**

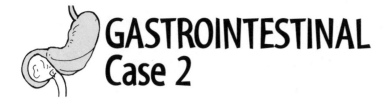

GASTROINTESTINAL Case 2

Mark, a 44-year-old farmer, visits his GP complaining of a short history of intermittent epigastric pain associated with heartburn and nausea.

List 6 pieces of lifestyle advice to help reduce his dyspepsia   *3 marks*

1. Lose weight.

2. Stop smoking.

3. Reduce alcohol.

4. Avoid large meals; take regular small meals.

5. Avoid eating near to bedtime.

6. Avoid foods that worsen symptoms.

7. Avoid non-steroidal anti-inflammatory drugs (NSAIDs).

8. Raise bed-head at night, eg prop head of bed up on books.

9. Avoid wearing tight clothes.

What drug should be initially prescribed to provide symptomatic relief?   *1 mark*

1. Antacid: to neutralise HCl.

2. Alginate compounds, eg Gaviscon: contain antacid + alginate compounds that float on the surface of stomach contents, reducing reflux and protecting the oesophagus.

Mark returns a few weeks later, complaining of a worsening of his symptoms.

QUESTIONS
PAGES 37–40

List 4 symptoms that would warrant further investigation   *2 marks*

1. Persistent symptoms (> 4 weeks).

2. Symptoms not relieved by proton pump inhibitors (PPI).

3. Weight loss.

4. Haematemesis.

5. Repeated vomiting.

6. Melaena.

7. Dysphagia.

List 6 causes of dysphagia   *3 marks*

ⓘ The causes of dysphagia can be classified as (1) extrinsic, (2) intrinsic and (3) motility disorders.

1. Extrinsic: **lung cancer, goitre, mediastinal lymph nodes.**

2. Intrinsic: **foreign body, benign stricture, malignant stricture (ie oesophageal cancer), pharyngeal pouch, oesophageal ring (narrowing of proximal end of oesophagus), oesophageal web (associated with iron-deficiency anaemia), oesophagitis, oesophageal candidiasis.**

3. Motility disorders: **achalasia, bulbar palsy, pseudobulbar palsy, myasthenia gravis, systemic sclerosis.**

List 3 procedures that may be used to investigate his symptoms   *3 marks*

1. Upper gastrointestinal (GI) endoscopy (oesophago-gastro-duodenoscopy, OGD): used to exclude organic causes of dyspepsia.

2. pH monitoring: 24-hour monitoring using a probe positioned in the lower oesphagus to assess the number of reflux episodes, to confirm gastro-oesophageal reflux disease (GORD).

3. Barium meal: may show hiatus hernia (a cause of GORD), with or without barium reflux.

Name 4 complications of GORD **2 marks**

1. Oesophagitis.

2. Ulceration: this may cause haematemesis or anaemia.

3. Benign oesophageal stricture: this may cause dysphagia.

4. Barrett's oesophagus: this is a pre-malignant change in the oesophageal mucosa, with the squamocolumnar junction (z line) migrating upwards.

Mark's GP arranges an outpatient appointment for him to undergo OGD, which diagnoses oesophagitis.

What drug may be prescribed to treat his oesophagitis? **1 mark**

1. H₂ antagonist, eg ranitidine (Zantac).

2. Proton pump inhibitor (PPI), eg omeprazole (Losec), lansoprazole (Zoton).

🛈 For OGD-confirmed oesophagitis, give an H2 antagonist; consider PPI for severe symptoms (with or without ulceration, Barrett's oesophagus, stricture). Also consider prokinetic drugs (eg metoclopramide, domperidone), which increase gastric emptying.

In another patient with rheumatoid arthritis receiving long-term NSAID therapy, a gastric ulcer is diagnosed on OGD. The two main causes of peptic ulcer disease are NSAIDs and Helicobacter pylori infection. H. pylori infection is detected by positive serology or ¹³C-urea breath test and eradicated by a 1-week triple therapy regimen.

What does this regimen involve? **1 mark**

This involves 1 week of treatment with:

1. PPI.

2. Amoxicillin.

3. Clarithromycin or metronidazole.

🛈 This achieves eradication in > 90% of cases and usually requires no further antisecretory treatment.

List 2 other complications of NSAIDs   *1 mark*

1. Asthma attack: NSAIDs, in particular aspirin, can trigger an acute asthma attack by triggering histamine release.

2. Renal failure (both acute and chronic renal failure): by reducing renal perfusion and tubulointerstitial nephritis.

3. Fluid overload as a result of inhibition of prostaglandin-mediated inhibition of Na$^+$ reabsorption.

4. Bleeding: aspirin, via its antiplatelet activity, may cause haemorrhage.

Name 2 drugs used to reduce the GI side-effects of NSAIDs   *1 mark*

NSAIDs inhibit cyclo-oxygenase (COX), which exists in two isoforms: COX1 is constitutively expressed in many tissues, and inhibition causes loss of gastric mucosal protection; COX2 is induced in response to inflammation. GI side-effects can be reduced by:

1. Selective COX2 inhibitor, eg rofecoxib.

2. Non-selective NSAID + PPI.

3. Non-selective NSAID + misoprostol (prostaglandin analogue).

🛈 However, there is no evidence that COX2 + gastroprotective drug further reduces GI side-effects.

List 4 causes of anaemia in rheumatoid arthritis   *2 marks*

1. Anaemia of chronic disease.

2. NSAID-induced GI bleeds.

3. Disease-modifying-drug-induced bone marrow suppression.

4. Hypersplenism associated with Felty's syndrome.

5. Pernicious anaemia: autoimmune disease associated with rheumatoid arthritis.

6. Haemolysis (drug induced by sulfalazine or dapsone).

Total: *20 marks*

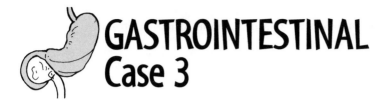

GASTROINTESTINAL
Case 3

*Nick, a mountain guide, is admitted to hospital by his GP,
complaining of malaise, anorexia and right upper quadrant pain. On
examination he is jaundiced and has a palpably enlarged smooth
liver and ascites.*

List 3 other <u>abdominal</u> signs of liver disease   **3 marks**

1. Splenomegaly: due to portal hypertension.

**2. Caput medusa (dilated collateral veins around the umbilicus): due to portal
hypertension.**

3. Skin bruising (due to abnormal coagulation).

4. Scratch marks: due to bile-salt pruritus.

🛈 Other signs of liver disease include: hands (clubbing, palmar erythema,
leuconychia, Dupuytren's contracture), endocrine disturbances (loss of
body hair, testicular atrophy, gynaecomastia), hepatic fetor and hand flap
(features of hepatic encephalopathy), peripheral oedema (as a result of
hypoalbuminaemia), and spider naevi (occur on upper body in the
drainage of the superior vena cava).

List 4 conditions that may cause ascites   **2 marks**

**Ascites is free fluid in the peritoneal cavity and can be demonstrated by shifting
dullness or a fluid thrill. Causes of ascites include:**

1. Malignancy of any intra-abdominal organ, eg ovarian cancer.

2. Liver cirrhosis (most common cause).

3. Pancreatitis.

QUESTIONS
PAGES 41–44

183

4. **Hypoalbuminaemia, eg in nephropathy, protein-losing enteropathy, malnutrition.**

5. **Heart failure.**

6. **Constrictive pericarditis.**

7. **Hepatic vein obstruction (Budd-Chiari syndrome), eg due to a thrombosis, tumour.**

8. **Hypothyroidism.**

9. **Tuberculosis infection.**

List 4 risk factors for jaundice that you would enquire about in the social history

2 marks

1. **Recent travel abroad: to areas endemic for hepatitis A virus.**

2. **Intravenous drug use: increased risk of hepatitis B virus (HBV) and hepatitis C virus (HCV).**

3. **Tattoos: increased risk of HBV and HCV.**

4. **Excessive alcohol consumption: alcoholic liver disease.**

5. **Homosexuality: increased risk of HBV.**

6. **Healthcare worker: increased risk of HBV and HCV.**

7. **Farm or sewage worker: increased risk of *Leptospira* infection.**

8. **Water sports: increased risk of *Leptospira* infection.**

Several blood tests are requested, to assess the severity of Nick's liver disease.

Name 2 blood tests used to assess liver synthetic function   *2 marks*

1. **Albumin (35–50 g/l): decreased in chronic liver disease.**

2. **International normalised ratio (INR, 0.9–1.2) or prothrombin time (10–14 s): increased in both acute and chronic liver disease.**

Gastrointestinal

ⓘ Other blood tests used to assess severity of liver disease are full blood count (decreased white cell count and decreased platelets with hypersplenism), urea and electrolytes (may get decreased Na$^+$ with severe cirrhosis), liver function tests (LFT; may get increased aspartate aminotransferase (AST), alanine aminotransferase (ALT), alkaline phosphatase (ALP), γ-glutamyl transpeptidase (γGT) and bilirubin).

List 4 extrahepatic causes of the following LFT profile: AST 14 iu/l, ALT 21 iu/l, ALP 270 iu/l, γGT 177 iu/l, bilirubin 102 µmol/l   *2 marks*

The LFT profile shows hyperbilirubinaemia (normal range 3–17 µmol/l) with increased ALP (30–150 iu/l) and γGT (11–51 iu/l) and normal ALT and AST (3–35 iu/l), which is associated with both intra- and extrahepatic cholestasis. Extrahepatic causes of cholestasis include:

1. Gallstones in the common bile duct.

2. Cancer in the head of the pancreas.

3. Pancreatitis.

4. Benign stricture of the common bile duct, eg complication of endoscopic retrograde cholangiopancreatography.

5. Sclerosing cholangitis, eg associated with inflammatory bowel disease.

6. Cholangiocarcinoma.

Ultrasound scan reveals an enlarged liver, with hepatic changes consistent with cirrhosis.

In the absence of obvious risk factors, list 3 blood tests you would request to identify the cause of Nick's cirrhosis   *3 marks*

1. HBV and HCV serology.

2. alpha-1-antitrypsin concentration: to exclude alpha-1-antitrypsin deficiency.

3. **Copper studies (decreased copper and caeruloplasmin, a copper-containing protein synthesised by the liver): to exclude Wilson's disease resulting in copper deposition in the liver.**

4. **Iron studies (increased iron and ferritin; decreased total iron-binding capacity): to exclude haemochromatosis resulting in iron deposition in the liver.**

5. **Autoantibodies: used to identify autoimmune causes of cirrhosis. Anti-mitochondrial antibody (primary biliary cirrhosis), anti-nuclear antibody and smooth muscle antibody (autoimmune hepatitis).**

Liver cirrhosis is confirmed by liver biopsy showing micronodular cirrhosis.

What is the most likely cause of Nick's cirrhosis?　　　　　*1 mark*

1. Alcohol.

ⓘ The major causes of cirrhosis are alcohol and chronic HBV and HCV infection. On biopsy, alcoholic cirrhosis is associated with micronodular cirrhosis (as is biliary cirrhosis) and viral infection with macronodular cirrhosis.

Two days later Nick's condition starts to deteriorate, and he complains of severe abdominal pain. On examination, his abdomen is very tender with guarding and he is pyrexial.

What is the likely complication?　　　　　*2 mark*

1. Bacterial peritonitis.

ⓘ Spontaneous bacterial peritonitis is a serious complication affecting approximately 10% of cirrhosis patients with ascites. It should be suspected in any patient with clinical deterioration, even in the absence of abdominal pain and pyrexia. It is treated with broad-spectrum antibiotics, eg cephalosporin and metronidazole.

How would you confirm your diagnosis? *1 mark*

1. Aspirate ascitic fluid for microscopy, culture and sensitivities.

🛈 A white cell count > 250/mm³ in aspirated ascitic fluid is considered diagnostic of bacterial peritonitis.

List 4 other complications of cirrhosis *2 marks*

1. Hepatocellular carcinoma: screen by regular ultrasound scan and α-fetoprotein.

2. Renal failure (hepatorenal syndrome).

3. Hepatic encephalopathy: due to blood bypassing the liver by portosystemic collaterals, causing neurotoxicity, eg confusion.

4. Portal hypertension: causes gastrointestinal haemorrhage (see Gastrointestinal Case 1), hypersplenism.

Total: *20 marks*

Gastrointestinal

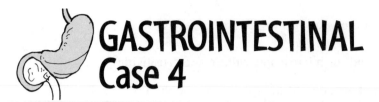

GASTROINTESTINAL
Case 4

Freda, a 64-year-old lady, presents to A&E with severe sudden-onset right subcostal pain. She also complains of nausea, vomiting and sweating. On examination she has a temperature of 38.4 °C and is tachycardic.

List 6 differential diagnoses   **3 marks**

1. Acute cholecystitis.

2. Biliary colic.

3. Cholangitis.

4. Peptic ulcer disease/perforation.

5. Hepatitis.

6. Myocardial infarction.

7. Renal colic.

8. Right basal pneumonia.

9. Appendicitis (high-lying).

10. Acute pancreatitis.

On examination, you find a positive Murphy's sign.

What is your likely diagnosis?   **1 mark**

1. Acute cholecystitis.

QUESTIONS
PAGES 45–50

Gastrointestinal

ℹ Murphy's sign is arrest of inspiration (because of severe pain) on palpation just below the right subcostal margin, due to the inflamed gallbladder descending to touch your hand (only positive if the same test on the left-hand side is negative).

ℹ Murphy's sign is associated with acute cholecystitis. Acute cholecystitis is caused by gallstones obstructing the cystic duct, causing distension of the gallbladder (which may cause local peritonism) and (sterile) inflammation (increased white cell count, fever). Presenting symptoms include severe right upper quadrant pain with nausea, vomiting and sweating.

Freda's ultrasound scan (USS) is shown:

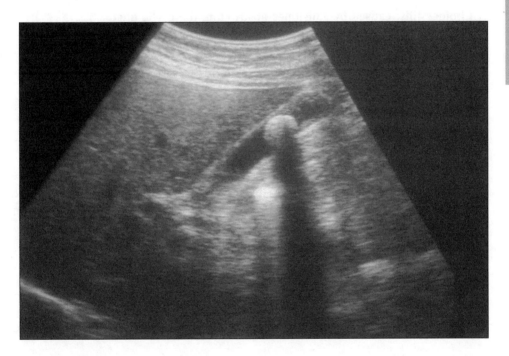

List 4 features on the USS that confirm your diagnosis **4 marks**

1. Presence of gallstones.

2. Biliary sludge.

3. Thickened gallbladder wall.

4. Distension of the gallbladder.

5. Free fluid around the gallbladder (pericholecystic fluid).

Freda is initially managed by a nil-by-mouth regimen, iv fluids, antiemetic, im pethidine and prophylactic antibiotics, and she appears to settle on this conservative regimen. She is scheduled for elective cholecystectomy later that week.

Name 6 complications of gallstones   *3 marks*

1. Biliary colic: caused by bile duct attempting to shift impacted gallstones.

2. Cholecystitis: caused by gallstones obstructing the cystic duct.

3. Acute pancreatitis.

4. Empyema: obstructed gallbladder fills with pus.

5. Obstructive jaundice: caused by gallstones obstructing the common bile duct.

6. Cholangitis: infection of the bile ducts causing right upper quadrant pain, jaundice and rigors.

7. Gall bladder perforation and generalised peritonitis.

8. Gall stone ileus: caused by gallstones obstructing the small bowel.

ⓘ The majority of patients with cholecystitis improve on conservative management with cholecystectomy to prevent recurrence. Ideally, this should be performed within days of an acute attack (though alternatively it may be performed 2–3 months later). Signs of complications require immediate surgery.

The next day, however, Freda experiences severe central abdominal pain radiating to her back and vomiting, and appears jaundiced. Her blood test shows an increased serum amylase concentration of 1650 units/dl.

What is the likely complication? *1 mark*

1. She has developed acute pancreatitis.

🛈 Gallstones and alcohol are the two most common causes of acute pancreatitis. Gallstones can cause acute pancreatitis by blocking the hepatopancreatic ampulla, causing reflux back up the main pancreatic duct and leading to pancreatic autodigestion.

Name 4 other causes of increased serum amylase *2 marks*

Serum amylase is increased in any cause of an acute abdomen. It is <u>only</u> diagnostic of acute pancreatitis if serum concentrations are > 1000 units/dl – ie 5 x the normal upper limit of < 180 units/dl. Below are several examples of an acute abdomen (see above also):

1. Pelvic inflammatory disease.

2. Ruptured ectopic pregnancy.

3. Ovarian cyst rupture.

4. Inflammatory bowel disease.

5. Diverticulitis.

6. Bowel obstruction.

7. Perforated bowel.

8. Ruptured abdominal aortic aneurysm.

9. Diabetic ketoacidosis.

List 6 blood variables used to assess the severity of her condition   *3 marks*

Variable	Positive value	Normal range
WCC ($\times$ 10⁹/l)	> 15	4–11
Blood glucose (mmol/l)	> 10	4–6
Albumin (g/l)	< 32	35–50
Urea (mmol/l)	> 16	2.5–6.7
AST (units/l)	> 100	3–35
Calcium (mmol/l)	< 2	2.12–2.65
LDH (iu/l)	> 600	70–250
paO$_2$ (kPa)	< 8	10–12

(WCC = white cell count, AST = aspartate aminotransferase, LDH = lactate dehydrogenase, paO$_2$ = arterial partial pressure of oxygen)

🛈 The Glasgow scoring system is used to predict the severity of acute pancreatitis from both gallstones and alcohol (Ranson's criterion is valid for alcohol-induced pancreatitis only). Age > 55 years is also considered. Three or more positive criteria indicates severe disease (associated with 50% mortality).

On examination, Freda shows signs of hypovolaemic shock and is given high-flow O$_2$ and iv saline.

List 6 signs indicating hypovolaemic shock   *3 marks*

1. Systolic blood pressure < 90 mmHg (though this may be a late sign as a result of a compensatory increase in peripheral resistance).

2. Tachycardia, ie heart rate > 100 bpm.

3. Increased capillary refill time, ie > 2 s.

4. Cold peripheries.

5. Oliguria, anuria (as a result of renal hypoperfusion).

6. Confusion (as a result of cerebral hypoperfusion).

7. Hyperventilation (as a result of metabolic acidosis).

🔵 Shock is a physiological state characterised by a significant, systemic reduction in tissue perfusion. In simple terms, shock is present when the heart rate value is higher than the systolic blood pressure. Pancreatitis can cause hypovolaemic shock as a result of collection of fluid in the peripancreatic region (termed third-space loss). This is treated with O_2 and iv fluids (saline or colloids titrated against blood pressure and urine output).

In fluid therapy, what minimum urinary output do you aim for?   *1 mark*

1. Aim for urine flow > 30 ml/h (ideally, should be 60 ml/h).

Give 2 complications of fluid overload   *1 mark*

1. Cardiac failure, causing pulmonary oedema.

2. Non-cardiogenic pulmonary oedema.

3. Peripheral oedema.

🔵 Fluid overload can cause cardiac dilatation, leading to a reduction in stroke volume resulting in cardiac failure. This may increase the pressure in the left atrium, which can subsequently cause pulmonary oedema.

What are the normal daily sodium and potassium requirements?   *2 marks*

1. Na$^+$: 100–150 mmol (1.5–2 mmol/kg body weight).

2. K$^+$: 60 mmol (1 mmol/kg body weight).

Freda remains hypotensive despite adequate fluid treatment.

What class of drug would you give Freda?   *1 mark*

1. Inotropes, eg dopamine, dobutamine, adrenaline, noradrenaline.

🔵 If the signs of shock persist despite adequate fluid replacement, inotropic agents must be given, to improve cardiac output and blood pressure thus ensuring adequate perfusion of vital organs.

She is resuscitated on this treatment.

What is the recommended procedure for her condition within the first 72 hours?

1 mark

1. Endoscopic retrograde cholangiopancreatography (ERCP), with or without sphincterotomy and removal of any stones.

ℹ ERCP involves insertion of an endoscope into the second part of the duodenum, cannulating the ampulla and injecting radio-opaque dye to visualise the biliary tree (an alternative imaging technique is magnetic resonance cholangiopancreatography). Any stone found on X-ray can be removed by sphincterotomy of the biliary sphincter and swept clear.

Freda undergoes a cholecystectomy before discharge.

List 2 advantages each of laparoscopic and open cholecystectomy   *2 marks*

1. Laparoscopic: **reduced wound pain, less scar formation, shorter inpatient stay/quicker recovery.**

1. Open: **lower risk of bile-duct injury, lower risk of damage to adjacent structures, any stones in the common bile duct can be removed at the same time, technically easier.**

Give 4 complications of cholecystectomy   *2 marks*

1. Death: fewer than 1 per 1000.

2. Bile-duct injury.

3. Bile leakage.

4. Jaundice caused by retained ductal stones (can be removed by ERCP).

5. Wound infection.

6. General complications of any surgical procedure, eg pulmonary embolism, chest infection.

Total: *30 marks*

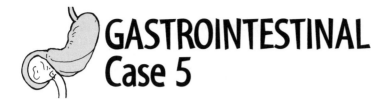

GASTROINTESTINAL
Case 5

Annie, a 25-year-old physiotherapist, presents with a 4-week history of diarrhoea with some mucus and blood mixed in her stool. She also complains of general abdominal discomfort, malaise and weight loss.

List 6 differential diagnoses of weight loss other than malignancy   ***3 marks***

1. Inflammatory bowel disease.

2. Malabsorption, eg coeliac disease, pancreatic insufficiency.

3. Chronic respiratory disease.

4. Hyperthyroidism.

5. Diabetes mellitus.

6. Addison's disease.

7. Chronic infection, eg tuberculosis, human immunodeficiency virus.

8. Psychiatric, eg depression, anorexia nervosa.

List 6 causes of bloody diarrhoea   ***3 marks***

1. Ulcerative colitis.

2. Crohn's disease.

3. Colorectal cancer.

4. Colonic polyps.

5. Ischaemic colitis: due to acute or chronic ischaemia of the bowel.

QUESTIONS
PAGES 51–54

195

6. Pseudomembranous colitis: caused by overgrowth of *Clostridium difficile* after antibiotic therapy.

7. Infective (dysentery): *Escherichia coli, Shigella, Salmonella, Campylobacter.*

Why would you do a plain abdominal X-ray in an acute attack of ulcerative colitis? *2 marks*

1. To exclude toxic dilatation, ie colon diameter > 5 cm, which is associated with a high risk of perforation.

Other investigations for ulcerative colitis include: full blood count (anaemia), vitamin B12 and folate (often low if terminal ileitis present), urea and electrolytes (electrolyte imbalance due to diarrhoea), liver function tests (may be deranged, albumin often low), erythrocyte sedimentation rate/C-reactive protein (severity of inflammation), stool and blood microscopy, culture and sensitivities (to exclude infectious diarrhoea), and sigmoidoscopy. A barium enema or colonoscopy with biopsy to assess disease extent is contraindicated during an acute severe attack of ulcerative colitis.

Annie is sent for a sigmoidoscopy, which reveals a superficial continuous inflammation of the rectum. The mucosa looks reddened and inflamed, consistent with ulcerative colitis.

List 3 pathological differences between ulcerative colitis and Crohn's disease *3 marks*

1. Ulcerative colitis involves only the bowel mucosa, whereas Crohn's disease involves all layers of the bowel wall (transmural).

2. Crohn's disease causes skip lesions (normal areas of bowel in between).

3. Crohn's disease can affect any part of the gastrointestinal tract, but typically affects the terminal ileum and ascending colon.

4. Ulcerative colitis can affect the rectum alone (proctitis), but can also extend proximally to involve part or all of the colon (colitis); it rarely spreads proximally beyond the colon (termed backwash ileitis).

List 4 extra-intestinal manifestations of inflammatory bowel disease **2 marks**

Related to disease activity		Unrelated to disease activity	
Mouth	Aphthous ulcers	**Kidney**	Stones
Skin	Pyoderma gangrenosum, erythema nodosum	**Liver**	Sclerosing cholangitis, fatty changes, cirrhosis cholangiocarcinoma
Eyes	Conjunctivitis, episcleritis, uveitis		
Joints	Monoarticular arthritis, ankylosing spondylitis	**Gallbladder**	Stones
		Hands	Clubbing

🛈 Extra-intestinal manifestations occur in 10–20% of patients.

List 6 features used to assess the severity of ulcerative colitis **3 marks**

Features	Mild	Moderate	Severe attack
Motions per day	< 4	4–6	> 6
Rectal bleeding	Little	Moderate	Large amounts
Temperature (°C)	Apyrexial	Intermediate	> 37.8
Heart rate (bpm)	< 70	70–90	> 90
Haemoglobin (g/dl)	> 11	10.5–11	< 10.5
ESR (mm/h)	Normal	Intermediate	> 30

(ESR = erythrocyte sedimentation rate)

🛈 Ulcerative colitis can be classified according to the above features as mild, moderate or severe, which is used to determine management. Mild and moderate attacks can be treated with rectal and oral steroids, respectively; severe attacks require admittance to hospital and treatment by a nil-by-mouth regimen, iv fluids + potassium supplements (also consider total parenteral nutrition), iv and rectal steroids and, if necessary, blood transfusion.

Annie is treated with oral prednisolone.

Give 8 complications of long-term oral steroid treatment   *4 marks*

1. Impaired glucose tolerance (may progress to diabetes mellitus).

2. Mental disturbance, eg euphoria, agitation or depression.

3. Osteoporosis (especially a risk in postmenopausal women).

4. Avascular necrosis of the femoral neck.

5. Cushing's syndrome: easy bruising, moon face, buffalo hump, striae.

6. Wasting and thinning of the skin.

7. Muscle wasting (proximal myopathy).

8. Hypertension.

9. Dyspepsia (may also cause peptic ulcer disease).

10. Cataracts.

11. Immune suppression increasing risk of infections.

🛈 Prolonged use of corticosteroids may also cause suppression of the hypothalamus–pituitary–adrenal (HPA) axis. Acute adrenal insufficiency (Addison's crisis) may develop if steroids are withdrawn too quickly or during physiological stress (eg surgery, trauma or illness). Therefore, in prolonged steroid treatment – ie > 3 weeks – steroids should be withdrawn slowly (to allow the HPA axis to recover) and the patient should carry a steroid treatment warning card.

What alternative can you prescribe in patients with severe steroid side-effects, to maintain remission and reduce steroid dose?   *2 marks*

1. Azathioprine.

 Azathioprine is an immunosuppressant. It can be used as a steroid-sparing agent in those with severe steroid side-effects or those with frequent relapses on withdrawal of steroids. Remission is also maintained on a 5-aminosalicylic acid agent, eg sulfasalazine or mesalazine. Surgery is curative of the intestinal features of ulcerative colitis and typically involves colectomy with an ileostomy or ileo-anal pouch reconstruction. Indications for surgery include perforation, massive haemorrhage, toxic dilatation and failure to respond to medication.

Give 3 complications of inflammatory bowel disease   *3 marks*

1. Perforation.

2. Bleeding: massive haemorrhage is rare.

3. Malnutrition.

4. Toxic dilatation of the colon: this may occur during an acute severe attack of ulcerative colitis (and Crohn's disease). This should be expected in any patient developing abdominal distension and is diagnosed on abdominal X-ray by a colon diameter > 5 cm. In the absence of a response to high-dose steroids, emergency surgery may be required, as the risk of perforation is high.

5. Colon cancer: incidence of colon cancer is increased in ulcerative colitis (and less so in Crohn's disease). Risk is greatest in those with extensive ulcerative colitis for more than 10 years.

Total: *25 marks*

Gastrointestinal

NEUROLOGICAL CASES:
ANSWERS

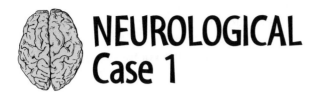

NEUROLOGICAL Case 1

Simon, a 72-year-old retired chiropractor, is found collapsed at home with sudden onset hemiparesis without loss of consciousness. Examination reveals signs of an upper motor neurone lesion, sensory loss and homonymous hemianopia on the affected side.

Indicate at '?' the expected findings according to the type of lesion **4 marks**

	UMN lesion	LMN lesion
Reflexes	Hyperreflexia ± clonus	Reduced or absent reflexes
Tone	Spastic (though initially after a CVA may be hypotonic)	Hypotonic
Plantars	Extensor (or upgoing)	Flexor (or downgoing)
Muscle bulk	Normal (no fasciculation)	Wasted (takes approximately 2 weeks to show signs of muscle wasting) with fasciculation

(UMN = upper motor neurone, LMN = lower motor neurone)

Name 2 sensory modalities carried in the posterior column **2 marks**

1. Proprioception.

2. Vibration.

3. Discriminative touch.

ⓘ Two major ascending pathways are involved in somatic sensory perception: (1) posterior column–medial lemniscal pathway; (2) spinothalamic pathway carrying pain, temperature and light touch.

QUESTIONS
PAGES 57–60

List 2 visual symptoms Simon might be complaining of   **2 marks**

Homonymous hemianopia causes loss of vision in the contralateral visual field, causing patients to complain of:

1. Knocking into objects.

2. Seeing only half of objects, eg face, clock, plate of food.

3. Unable to read as sees only half the page.

🛈 Homonymous hemianopia is caused by lesions to the optic tract, optic radiation or visual cortex (macular vision may be spared) and may arise from occlusions to the middle cerebral artery (which supplies the optic radiation) or posterior cerebral artery (which supplies the occipital cortex).

Name 4 cardiac conditions that may cause an embolic cerebrovascular accident (CVA)   **2 marks**

A CVA may be caused by haemorrhage, thrombosis in situ, atherothrombo-embolism or a heart embolus:

1. Atrial fibrillation.

2. Myocardial infarction causing a mural thrombus.

3. Subacute bacterial endocarditis.

4. Aortic or mitral valve disease.

5. Patent foramen ovale (paradoxical embolus).

🛈 When examining a stroke patient, you need to identify the neurological deficits by carrying out a full neurological examination, identify factors that may cause complications, eg dysphagia, and identify likely causes of the stroke, eg full cardiovascular system examination to exclude atrial fibrillation, heart murmurs, carotid bruits.

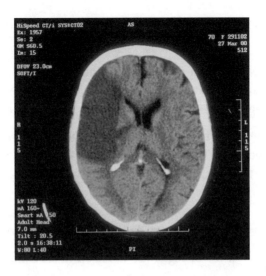

Simon's brain computed tomography scan is shown:

What cerebral artery is affected?   **2 marks**

1. Right (1 mark) middle cerebral artery (1 mark).

ⓘ The middle cerebral artery supplies the lateral surfaces of the cerebral hemispheres and the optic radiation (cortical branches), as well as supplying the internal capsule, corpus striatum and thalamus (central branches). A lesion to the middle cerebral artery at its origin causes contralateral hemiparesis and sensory loss, contralateral homonymous hemianopia, and dysphasia (if dominant hemisphere) or dyspraxia (if non-dominant hemisphere).

Is Simon's CVA caused by vascular occlusion or haemorrhage?   **1 mark**

1. Vascular occlusion.

ⓘ An infarct due to a vascular occlusion is visualised as a low-density area (ie black on computed tomography (CT) scan), with loss of grey/white matter differentiation. There is often a surrounding black area due to cerebral oedema. Haemorrhage initially appears as an area of increased density (ie white).

Neurological

List 6 features associated with a lesion to the vertebrobasilar territory   **3 marks**

In theory, clinical features of a CVA relate to the affected artery, though this is often complicated by collateral circulation. A lesion to the vertebrobasilar territory, which supplies the brainstem and cerebellum, may cause:

1. **Cranial nerve signs (due to brainstem lesion), eg diplopia (cranial nerves III, IV, VI), facial weakness (VII), facial numbness (V), vertigo (VIII), dysphagia (IX, X) and dysarthria (IX, X, XII).**

2. **Ataxia (due to lesion to cerebellum).**

3. **Weakness in both arms or legs (due to lesion to corticospinal tracts).**

4. **Sensory loss in both arms or legs (due to lesion to ascending sensory pathways).**

5. **Coma (due to lesion to reticular formation).**

6. **Locked-in syndrome, ie aware but unable to respond (due to massive brainstem lesion).**

7. **Lateral medullary syndrome, eg vertigo, ataxia, ipsilateral loss of pain and temperature on the face (due to posterior inferior cerebellar artery lesion).**

List 6 additional investigations you might consider, briefly explaining why

6 marks

1. **Full blood count (FBC): to exclude polycythaemia and thrombocytosis (increased risk of thrombosis).**

2. **Urea and electrolytes (U&Es): renal impairment may be due to, or a result of, hypertension.**

3. **Erythrocyte sedimentation rate (ESR): to exclude temporal arteritis.**

4. **Clotting screen: may indicate increased risk of thrombosis or haemorrhage.**

5. **Syphilis serology: to exclude neurosyphilis.**

6. **Glucose and lipids: secondary prevention of atherosclerosis.**

7. **Blood cultures: if subacute bacterial endocarditis is suspected.**

8. **Autoantibodies: to exclude systemic lupus erythematosus in younger patients (increased risk of thrombosis).**

9. **ECG: to exclude atrial fibrillation or myocardial infarction.**

10. **Echocardiogram: to exclude cardiac sources of emboli, eg mural thrombus.**

11. **Carotid Doppler: to exclude internal carotid artery stenosis.**

12. **Chest X-ray: to exclude lung cancer causing brain metastases (differential diagnosis).**

🛈 The above represents a comprehensive list of investigations. Initially, the following tests should be performed: FBC, U&Es, ESR, glucose, lipids, ECG and brain CT scan, with additional investigations where appropriate.

Name 6 health professionals involved in Simon's rehabilitation   *3 marks*

Rehabilitation of CVA patients involves a multidisciplinary approach:

1. **GP: to treat modifiable risk factors such as hypertension.**

2. **Dietician: to address any nutritional problems as a result of the stroke, eg dysphagia.**

3. **Physiotherapist: to help reduce spasticity.**

4. **Occupational therapist: to reduce functional disabilities.**

5. **Speech therapist: to treat any dysphagia, dysphasia, dysarthria.**

6. **Community nurse: to enable the patient to continue to live at home.**

7. **Social worker: to ensure the appropriate care package is in place.**

Total: *25 marks*

NEUROLOGICAL
Case 2

Mona, an 82-year-old widow, is brought into A&E after her carer found her, that afternoon, still in bed and more confused than normal. On examination she has a Glasgow Coma Scale score of 11/15 and a temperature of 38.5 °C; her blood pressure is 116/64 mmHg, her heart rate is 90 bpm and regular; the respiratory rate is 28/min and there is bronchial breathing at her right lung base.

List 6 causes of acute confusion (delirium)   **3 marks**

1. **Infection: in particular, urinary tract infection (UTI) and pneumonia. Rarely, meningitis and encephalitis.**

2. **Metabolic: hypoglycaemia, renal failure, liver failure, electrolyte imbalance eg hyponatraemia.**

3. **Drugs (and drug withdrawal): eg benzodiazepines, opiates, alcohol.**

4. **Hypoxia: respiratory or cardiac failure.**

5. **Myocardial infarction.**

6. **Intracranial lesion: eg space-occupying lesion, increased intracranial pressure, head injury (eg subdural haematoma), epilepsy, cerebrovascular accident.**

7. **Nutritional deficiency: vitamin B12, thiamine (B1).**

List 4 non-invasive investigations you would do   **2 marks**

1. **Chest X-ray: to exclude pneumonia, pulmonary oedema.**

2. **ECG: to exclude myocardial infarction.**

QUESTIONS
PAGES 61–63

Neurological

3. **Urine dipstick: to exclude UTI; if blood, nitrites or leukocytes suggest UTI, send for microscopy, culture and sensitivities.**

4. **Sputum for microscopy, culture and sensitivities (though sample may be difficult to obtain in a confused patient).**

Mona's blood test results are shown:

Hb	15.1 g/dl	CRP	145 mg/l	pH	7.41
MCV	85 fl			pO_2	7.6 kPa
Platelets	320 x 10⁹/l	Glucose	24.7 mmol/l	pCO_2	5.1 kPa
WCC	21 x 10⁹/l			HCO_3^-	24 mmol/l
	(neutrophilia)	Bilirubin	12 μmol/l		
Na⁺	149 mmol/l	ALT	14 iu/l	Blood	Negative
K⁺	4.6 mmol/l	AST	12 iu/l	culture	
Urea	28.4 mmol/l	ALP	66 iu/l		
Creatinine	240 mmol/l				

(Hb = haemoglobin, MCV = mean cell volume, WCC = white cell count, CRP = C-reactive protein, ALT = alanine aminotransferase, AST = aspartate aminotransferase, ALP = alkaline phosphatase, pO_2, pCO_2 = partial pressures of oxygen and carbon dioxide, HCO_3^- = bicarbonate)

List 5 diagnoses inferred from these blood results **5 marks**

1. **Type I respiratory failure: decreased pO_2 with normal pCO_2.**

2. **Dehydration: increased sodium (normal range 135–145 mmol/l).**

3. **Renal impairment: increased urea (normal range 2.5–6.7 mmol/l) and creatinine (normal range 70–120 mmol/l).**

4. **Underlying infection: increased CRP (normal range < 10 mg/l), increased WCC (normal range 4–11 x 10⁹/l; neutrophilia suggests bacterial infection).**

5. **Hyperglycaemia: increased glucose (normal range 4–11 mmol/l).**

🛈 In Mona's case, the underlying cause of these abnormal blood results (and her acute confusion) is pneumonia (as indicated by increased CRP/WCC and consolidation on chest examination confirmed on chest X-ray) causing type I respiratory failure, dehydration causing hypernatraemia and acute renal failure, and transitory hyperglycaemia (even in the absence of underlying diabetes mellitus).

Neurological

List 4 causes of hyponatraemia   **4 marks**

The causes of hyponatraemia can be classified as due to increased extracellular fluid (ECF) (dilutional effect) or decreased ECF (where sodium loss is greater than fluid loss):

1. **Increased ECF: eg heart failure, hypoproteinaemia (eg cirrhosis, malabsorption), oliguric renal failure, syndrome of inappropriate antidiuretic hormone secretion (SIADH), water excess (eg excessive iv 5% dextrose), drugs (eg non-steroidal anti-inflammatory drugs, which promote water retention).**

2. **Decreased ECF: eg Addison's disease (aldosterone insufficiency), diarrhoea and vomiting, heat exposure, osmotic diuresis, eg diabetes mellitus, diuretic excess, diuretic stage of acute renal failure.**

ⓘ Note that, conversely, decreased ECF may also cause hypernatraemia when fluid loss is greater than sodium loss.

A diagnosis of pneumonia is made and Mona is successfully treated with iv cefuroxime and clarithromycin, sliding-scale insulin and iv fluids (0.9% saline). Before she is discharged from hospital, her underlying dementia is assessed and she records a Mini-Mental State Examination (MMSE) score of 18.

What MMSE score supports a diagnosis of dementia?   **1 mark**

1. MMSE < 25 supports a diagnosis of dementia.

ⓘ MMSE is scored out of 30: scores of 28–30 do not support a diagnosis of dementia. A score of 25–27 is borderline; < 25 supports a diagnosis of dementia (chronic confusion) in the absence of acute confusion and depression.

What are the 2 most common causes of dementia?   **1 mark**

1. Alzheimer's disease.

2. Vascular/multi-infarct dementia.

List 4 blood tests you would do to exclude treatable causes of dementia **4 marks**

Treatable causes of dementia include: hypothyroidism, tertiary syphilis, deficiency in vitamin B12, thiamine (B1) and folate, chronic alcohol abuse (eg cerebral atrophy, Wernicke-Korsakoff syndrome) and subdural haematoma.

1. Thyroid function tests.

2. Syphilis serology.

3. Liver function tests: alcohol abuse causes increased γ-glutamyl transferase.

4. Full blood count: macrocytic anaemia may suggest B12 or folate deficiency; macrocytosis without anaemia is a marker of alcohol abuse.

5. Vitamin B12, thiamine (B1) and folate concentrations.

Total: **20 marks**

Neurological

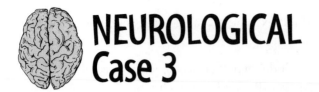 # NEUROLOGICAL Case 3

While on summer camp in the Brecon Beacons, 17-year-old Meriel is taken ill, complaining of headache, stiff neck and photophobia. Her teachers, worried she may have meningitis, rush her to the nearest A&E department.

Name 2 signs associated with meningeal irritation and briefly describe how they are elicited **2 marks**

1. **Kernig's sign: on lying supine with the knees and hips flexed, there is back pain on extending the knees.**

2. **Brudzinski's sign: on lying supine, flexion of the neck causes flexion of the hips and knees.**

If positive, these signs confirm irritation of the meninges, which occurs in meningitis. Similarly, flexing the neck to assess any resistance to movement or associated pain also suggests meningeal irritation (though local infections and arthritis of the spine may also cause neck stiffness).

A lumbar puncture to confirm the diagnosis is requested and Meriel is examined to exclude increased intracranial pressure (ICP).

List 4 causes of increased ICP **2 marks**

1. **Brain tumours: primary or secondary.**

2. **Head injury.**

3. **Intracranial haemorrhage, eg subarachnoid haemorrhage, subdural or extradural haematoma, intracerebral haemorrhage.**

4. **Infection, eg meningitis, encephalitis, abscess.**

QUESTIONS
PAGES 64–66

5. Hydrocephalus.

6. Status epilepticus (due to hypoxic oedema).

Give 6 signs in Meriel that indicate increased ICP   *3 marks*

1. Drowsiness, confusion, decreased consciousness.

2. Severe headache.

3. Irritability.

4. Fits/seizures.

5. Vomiting.

6. Bradycardia.

7. Increased blood pressure (Cushing's response).

8. False localising signs, eg cranial nerve (CN) III and VI palsies.

9. Irregular respiration, eg Cheyne-Stokes respiration (alternating hyperventilation and apnoea).

10. Papilloedema (late sign) or absence of venous pulsation at the optic disc.

11. Opisthotonus, ie arching of back and neck.

🛈 In infants, additional signs include bulging fontanelle and enlarged head circumference.

Describe what the eye would look like in a complete CN III palsy   *3 marks*

Increased ICP can, rarely, cause an ipsilateral CN III lesion (an example of a false localising sign):

1. Ptosis: as a result of levator palpebrae superioris (upper eyelid) paralysis.

2. The eye is deviated 'down and out': due to unopposed lateral rectus and superior oblique action.

3. The pupil is dilated and non-reactive: due to loss of parasympathetic innervation.

ⓘ Increased ICP can cause tentorial herniation, ie herniation of the cerebral hemispheres through the tentorial hiatus of the cerebellar tentorium, causing compression of the midbrain (this may also cause coning of the brainstem through the foramen magnum). If this happens it may cause decreased conscious level (as a result of compression of the reticular formation in the brainstem), cardiorespiratory depression (due to compression of the medulla) and false localising signs, eg CN III and VI palsies (because of the long pathways of these cranial nerves).

Give 2 contraindications (other than increased ICP) to lumbar puncture **2 marks**

1. Impaired clotting, eg warfarin: may cause a haematoma, leading to spinal cord compression.

2. Thrombocytopenia (platelet count < 40 x 10⁹/l): as above.

3. Local infection near the site of the puncture: may introduce infection into the cerebrospinal fluid (CSF).

4. Septicaemia: as above.

5. Cardiorespiratory instability.

ⓘ Lumbar puncture is diagnostic in meningitis. However, it is only carried out if there are no signs of increased ICP (a computed tomography (CT) brain scan is normally done first, to exclude increased ICP). This is because increased ICP may cause coning of the medulla if the CSF pressure below this level is reduced by a lumbar puncture.

There are no signs of increased ICP (confirmed on CT scan of the head), and a lumbar puncture is performed.

Indicate (↑, → or ↓) at '?' the expected CSF changes in bacterial meningitis

2 marks

	Normal	Bacterial meningitis	Viral meningitis
Appearance	Clear	↓ (turbid)	→ (Clear)
WCC	0–5/mm³	↑↑ (200–300/mm³)	↑
Protein	0.2–0.4 g/l	↑ (0.5–2.0 g/l)	↑ or → (< 1.0 g/l)
Glucose	> 50% of blood glucose	↓ (< 50% of blood glucose)	↓ or →

(WCC = white cell count)

🔵 Other tests performed include: full blood count, urea and electrolytes, liver function tests, C-reactive protein, coagulation screen, blood glucose (to compare with CSF), culture blood and throat swabs for bacteria (preferably before antibiotics), rapid antigen test for meningitis organisms (on blood, urine or CSF).

Meriel is diagnosed with meningococcal meningitis, her CSF Gram staining confirming Neisseria meningitidis.

What colour does *Neisseria meningitidis* give with Gram stain?   *1 mark*

1. Pink: *Neisseria meningitidis* is a Gram-negative diplococci.

🔵 Causative organisms of meningitis vary with the patient's age. The most common are: in neonates, *Escherichia coli*, *Listeria monocytogenes* and ß-haemolytic streptococci; in children, *Haemophilus influenzae* (unless the child has been vaccinated), *Streptococcus pneumoniae* and *Neisseria meningitidis* (meningococcal); in teenagers and adults, *Neisseria meningitidis* and *Streptococcus pneumoniae*.

Which antibiotic would you prescribe?   *1 mark*

1. High-dose iv benzyl penicillin or cephalosporin, eg cefotaxime.

🔵 If meningitis is suspected but the organism is unknown, give high-dose cephalosporin, eg ceftriaxone 2 g bid or cefotaxime 2 g tds empirically. Give the first dose immediately and then perform lumbar puncture.

List 4 complications of bacterial meningitis   *2 marks*

1. Death: untreated acute bacterial meningitis is almost always fatal.

2. Mental retardation.

3. Sensorineural deafness.

4. Focal neurological lesions, eg cranial nerve palsies.

5. Epilepsy.

Neurological

6. Hydrocephalus: results from impaired resorption of CSF and may require a ventricular shunt.

What prophylaxis do you give to contacts of Meriel and what do you warn them about? **2 marks**

1. Rifampicin (600 mg twice daily for 2 days).

2. Warn them about pink-coloured tears and urine.

Total: **20 marks**

OBSTETRICS & GYNAECOLOGY CASES: ANSWERS

OBSTETRICS & GYNAECOLOGY Case 1

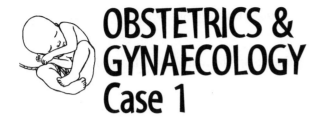

Sue, a 35-year-old primary school teacher, and her husband Peter, a 38-year-old salesman, are both delighted to discover that Sue is pregnant for the first time. Sue is now 10 weeks pregnant (her last menstrual period (LMP) was July 15 and her cycle is normally a regular 24 days) and she attends the antenatal clinic for her booking visit.

When is Sue's expected date of delivery (EDD)? *1 mark*

1. April 18

EDD = LMP (15 July) + 3 days (cycle length -21 days) + 9 months = 18 April (Naegele's rule)

List 6 blood tests you would offer *3 marks*

1. **Full blood count: to exclude anaemia (< 10.5 g/dl).**

2. **ABO group and Rhesus status: require ABO group if transfusions are required; if she is Rh-negative, offer anti-D-antigen prophylaxis (at 28 and 34 weeks) to prevent sensitisation.**

3. **Irregular red blood cell antibodies, eg anti-Kell antibodies: risk of haemolytic disease of the newborn (re-test at 28 weeks).**

4. **Rubella antibodies: ideally, screen before conception and, if negative, immunise (measles, mumps and rubella (MMR) vaccine is now the only vaccine available) and practice safe sex for at least 3 months. If negativity is only discovered at the booking visit, educate on importance of avoiding contact with infected individuals.**

QUESTIONS
PAGES 69–72

Obstetrics & Gynaecology

5. **Syphilis serology: it is necessary to exclude syphilis, which may cause congenital syphilis.**

6. **Hepatitis B virus (HBV): guidelines exist for managing HBV-positive women to prevent vertical transmission.**

7. **Human immunodeficiency virus (HIV): guidelines exist for managing HIV-positive women to prevent vertical transmission.**

🛈 There is no evidence that routine monitoring for gestational diabetes is effective and therefore it is not offered. Also offer urine tests for proteinuria (to exclude pre-eclampsia), culture (to exclude asymptomatic bacteriuria, which may cause pre-term birth) and ultrasound scan (USS) to determine gestational age (by crown–rump length or head circumference).

List 4 examples of dietary advice you would give Sue　　　　　*2 marks*

1. **Take folic acid 400 µg/day: this should ideally be taken before conception and during the first trimester, to reduce risks of neural tube defects (eg anencephaly, spina bifida).**

2. **Eat plenty of fruit and vegetables.**

3. **Avoid vitamin A supplementation (potentially teratogenic) and liver (which contains high concentrations of vitamin A).**

4. **Prevent *Listeria* infection (may cause mid-trimester miscarriage, pre-term labour, congenital listeriosis) by avoiding drinking unpasteurised milk, soft cheeses such as brie, pâté and any uncooked/undercooked meals.**

5. **Prevent *Toxoplasmosis* infection (may cause congenital abnormalities) by avoiding raw/undercooked meats such as steaks, and always washing hands after handling raw meat.**

6. **Prevent *Salmonella* infection (may cause neonatal septicaemia) by avoiding raw eggs, including mayonnaise and raw/undercooked meats, especially poultry.**

7. **Avoid alcohol in first trimester (may cause fetal alcohol syndrome) and limit intake to 1 unit/day thereafter.**

List 6 common minor symptoms of pregnancy Sue may experience   *3 marks*

1. **Nausea and vomiting: affects up to 75% of women. Typically worse during the first trimester.**

2. **Backache: common in late pregnancy. Felt over the sacroiliac joints, as a result of progesterone-mediated relaxation of ligaments and muscles.**

3. **Breathlessness: caused by progesterone-induced hyperventilation decreasing maternal $paCO_2$ so as to increase CO_2 exchange across the placenta.**

4. **Constipation: caused by progesterone-mediated reduced gut motility, exacerbated in late pregnancy by pressure of enlarged uterus.**

5. **Heartburn: caused by progesterone-mediated relaxation of lower oesophageal sphincter.**

6. **Varicose veins and haemorrhoids: caused by progesterone-mediated smooth muscle relaxation and venous obstruction due to the pregnant uterus.**

7. **Headaches, palpitations, fainting: as a result of changes in the cardiovascular system.**

8. **Urinary frequency: a result of pressure of fetal head on the bladder (need to exclude urinary tract infection).**

9. **Ankle oedema: due to fluid retention and mechanical obstruction preventing venous return.**

10. **Carpal tunnel syndrome: due to fluid retention.**

11. **Itching: common and may be due to pruritic eruption of pregnancy, ie an itchy papular rash. If generalised and severe, it is necessary to exclude cholestasis of pregnancy (a rare condition associated with intrauterine growth retardation (IUGR) and intrauterine death).**

Because of her age, Sue has an increased risk of chromosomal abnormalities, including Down's syndrome (her risk is 1 : 338).

Give an example (including what it measures) of a second trimester screening test for trisomy 21 **2 marks**

There are 2 tests used to screen for trisomy 21 in the second trimester (the arrows indicate the changes associated with trisomy 21):

1. Triple blood test: measures maternal serum alpha-fetoprotein (↓), human chorionic gonadotrophin (hCG) (↑) and unconjugated oestriol (↓).

2. Quadruple test: as triple test, plus inhibin A (↑).

ⓘ Screening for trisomy 21 in the first trimester involves: (1) nuchal translucency (USS measurement of the translucent subcutaneous space at the back of the neck of a fetus; > 3mm is associated with trisomy 21), (2) hCG, and (3) pregnancy-associated plasma protein A (↓); all three are collectively referred to as the 'combined test'. The 'integrated test' is the gold standard for detecting trisomy 21 and includes the combined test together with second-trimester screening; it has an 89% pick-up rate for a > 2% false-positive rate. Women with a positive screening test are offered a diagnostic test (eg amniocentesis, chorionic villi sampling).

At 28 weeks, Sue attends the antenatal clinic complaining of feeling tired and having fainted 2 days previously.

What 2 conditions should you exclude? **1 mark**

1. Anaemia: haemoglobin < 10.5 g/dl.

2. Postural hypotension: > 15 mmHg change in lying and standing systolic blood pressure.

How do you screen for pre-eclampsia? **1 mark**

1. Measure blood pressure and urine dipstick for proteinuria.

ⓘ Pre-eclampsia is pregnancy-induced hypertension, ie blood pressure ≥ 140/90 mmHg plus proteinuria with or without oedema. It typically develops after week 20 and is caused by poor trophoblast invasion of the spiral arteries in early pregnancy, leading to decreased blood supply to the feto-placental unit. This in turn leads to release of circulating factors, causing alterations in endothelial cells and resulting in increased maternal blood pressure, proteinuria and IUGR. It is a multisystem disorder (affecting kidneys, liver, blood and fetus), which may progress to eclampsia (eg convulsions, death). There is no cure except to terminate the pregnancy and deliver the baby.

List 4 symptoms associated with pre-eclampsia   *2 marks*

1. Headaches.

2. Visual disturbance, eg blurring.

3. Nausea and vomiting.

4. Swelling of face, hands and feet.

5. Epigastric pain.

🛈 However, pre-eclampsia may also be asymptomatic, so regular screening is essential.

On obstetric examination, the midwife finds that the pubic symphysis (fundal) height is 24 cm.

Give 4 reasons why Sue may be small for dates   *2 marks*

1. Incorrect dates.

2. Intrauterine growth retardation.

3. Constitutionally small baby.

4. Oligohydramnios, ie reduced amniotic fluid.

🛈 Fundal height is an approximate measure of fetal growth and should give an estimation of gestational age in weeks, eg at 28 weeks fundal height should be 28 cm ± 3 cm.

Obstetrics & Gynaecology

List 4 causes of intrauterine growth retardation **4 marks**

Causes of IUGR can be classified as:

1. **Maternal causes, eg malnutrition, smoking, systemic disease (eg renal disease, anaemia).**

2. **Placental insufficiency, eg multiple gestation, antepartum haemorrhage, antiphospholipid syndrome (reduces utero-placental perfusion), inadequate trophoblastic invasion as seen in pre-eclampsia.**

3. **Fetal causes, eg infections (eg cytomegalovirus), congenital malformations, chromosomal abnormalities eg trisomy 18.**

🛈 When placental insufficiency has been the cause, ie the fetus is starved, brain growth (and hence head circumference) is relatively spared, at the expense of liver glycogen and fat stores (causing reduced abdominal circumference), and is termed asymmetrical IUGR. Pregnancies at risk of IUGR (eg previous IUGR, small for dates) can be assessed for intrauterine growth restriction and a decision made whether to continue the pregnancy or deliver the baby (eg on the basis of fetal monitoring, growth charts, umbilical artery blood flow and gestational age). Babies with IUGR have an increased risk of hypoxia and death (in utero and during labour), hypothermia, hypoglycaemia, jaundice as a result of polycythaemia (postnatally), and type 2 diabetes, hypertension and cardiovascular disease (in adulthood).

List 4 topics you want to discuss with Sue in her third trimester **4 marks**

1. **Signs of labour: painful contractions occurring at less than 10-minute intervals, show (blood/mucous plug) and rupture of amniotic membranes.**

2. **Birth plan: eg where does she want to have the baby: home or hospital?**

3. **Pain management during delivery, eg epidural.**

4. **How does she intend to feed the baby: outline the benefits of breast-feeding.**

5. **Local antenatal classes: to prepare for delivery and preparation for the postnatal period.**

6. **Future contraceptive plans; eg cannot use combined oral contraceptives if breast-feeding.**

Total: **25 marks**

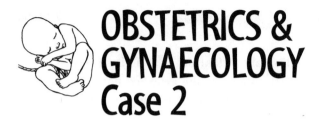

OBSTETRICS & GYNAECOLOGY
Case 2

26-year-old Debbie, 39 weeks pregnant with her first child, is out walking when her waters break. She is rushed to the labour ward by her husband Gerald and is complaining of regular painful contractions every 10 minutes.

List 4 questions you would ask   ***2 marks***

1. When is the baby due?

2. Have you felt the baby move?

3. Is it a single pregnancy or twins?

4. Are you aware of any problems with the pregnancy, eg malpresentation?

5. Is the liquor coloured (is there any meconium)?

6. Do you have any medical problems, eg diabetes mellitus?

7. Any problems with previous pregnancies, including delivery?

ⓘ The aim of these questions is to assess any risk to the baby and mother, eg if the baby is premature: previous poor pregnancy outcomes are risk factors for this pregnancy; passage of meconium may indicate that the fetus is distressed, but can be normal in a post-term pregnancy.

On obstetric palpation, fundal height is 40 cm, it is a cephalic presentation and the fetal head is engaged. On vaginal examination, the position is left occiput-lateral and the cervix is 4 cm dilated.

QUESTIONS
PAGES 73–76

Obstetrics & Gynaecology

List 6 <u>maternal</u> observations recorded on the partogram   *3 marks*

The partogram is a graphic record of labour that provides a visual record of cervical dilatation, enabling comparison against the expected norm and key maternal and fetal observations, thus allowing active management if required:

1. Heart rate, blood pressure and temperature.

2. Strength and frequency of contractions.

3. Cervical dilatation.

4. Urine volume: to exclude maternal dehydration.

5. Urine analysis, eg proteinuria, ketonuria.

6. iv infusions, eg oxytocin.

7. Any drugs, eg pethidine.

8. Liquor, ie colour of vaginal discharge.

🛈 Fetal observations include heart rate (normal range 110–150 bpm), position (displayed graphically), extent of fixing/engagement, station (relation of presenting part to ischial spines), moulding or caput.

Debbie's contractions become progressively more frequent and painful. Three hours later her cervical dilatation is reassessed and plotted on the partogram, demonstrating that Debbie's labour is progressing satisfactorily.

Give 2 examples each of non-pharmacological and pharmacological methods of pain relief   *2 marks*

1. Non-pharmacological (typically used during latent phase): **transcutaneous electrical nerve stimulation, back massage, relaxation and breathing exercises, warm bath.**

2. Pharmacological (typically used during active phase and stage 2): **nitric oxide + O_2 (gas and air), pethidine, epidural, spinal block.**

By how many centimetres should the cervix be dilated now?   *1 mark*

1. 7 cm, ie an increase of 3 cm above last recording, 3 hours ago, of 4 cm.

ⓘ Progress in the active phase (of the first stage of labour) is assessed by cervical dilatation from 3 cm to fully dilated (10 cm) and effaced. Dilatation typically proceeds at 1 cm/h in a primigravida and 2 cm/h in a multigravida.

List 4 causes of failure to progress in the first stage of labour   *2 marks*

1. Inefficient uterine contractions.

2. Malpresentation, eg face presentation, breech.

3. Malposition, eg occiput-posterior.

4. Cephalo–pelvic disproportion (CPD): disproportion between the fetal head and maternal pelvis.

5. Cervical dystocia: failure of cervical dilatation (eg due to previous trauma, surgery).

ⓘ Primary dysfunctional labour is slow progress during the active phase of labour (usually as a result of inefficient contractions). Secondary arrest is initial satisfactory progress followed by arrest after 7 cm dilatation (usually caused by CPD or malposition). Causes of delay in the second stage of labour (which should last less than 1 hour in a primigravida) include CPD (preventing internal rotation, termed deep transverse arrest), occiput-posterior position, secondary uterine inertia, maternal exhaustion, pain and anxiety.

During labour, Debbie's baby is intermittently monitored by cardiotocography (CTG) to assess whether her baby is distressed.

What 4 components are used to interpret a CTG?   *2 marks*

CTG monitors fetal heart rate alongside uterine contractions and is used in labour to detect fetal hypoxia (supported by passage of fresh meconium and scalp pH < 7.2). The 4 components used in interpreting a CTG are:

1. **Baseline heart rate: should be 110–150 bpm (abnormal if < 100 or > 170 bpm).**

2. **Baseline variability: baseline heart rate should vary between 6 and 15 bpm (abnormal if varies < 5 bpm over a 20-minute period).**

3. **Accelerations: defined as increase in heart rate of ≥ 15 bpm for ≥ 15 s in response to uterine activity. Should be ≥ 2 accelerations every 20 minutes (abnormal if none).**

4. **Decelerations: defined as decrease in heart rate of ≥ 15 bpm for ≥ 15 s in response to uterine activity. If early (ie trough of deceleration coincides with peak of contraction), they are considered normal in the late first stage of labour and the second stage. If late or variable, they are considered abnormal.**

🛈 If CTG is abnormal, lie the mother on her side (to avoid compression of vena cava), stop any oxytocin infusion and take a fetal scalp blood sample. If the pH is < 7.2 and/or there is fresh meconium, deliver immediately.

List 4 sequential stages in the passage of the fetus through the birth canal leading up to the delivery of the shoulders   *4 marks*

1. **Head engages, typically in occiput-transverse position.**

2. **Head descends further into the pelvis.**

3. **Head flexes onto chest so that presenting part is occiput or vertex.**

4. **Internal rotation (directed by the gutter-shaped pelvic floor) so that, typically, the occiput lies behind the pubic symphysis, ie anterior rotation.**

5. **Head extends from underneath the pubic symphysis, allowing the head to be delivered.**

6. **Restitution of the head so that it aligns with the obliquely placed shoulders.**

7. **External rotation so that the delivered head rotates to lie in a transverse position so that the shoulders lie in the anterior–posterior plane.**

This is followed by delivery of the anterior shoulder, followed by the posterior shoulder and, finally, by delivery of the rest of body.

Debbie delivers a pink and healthy boy, named Alex, who cries immediately.

List 4 steps in your immediate management of Alex   *2 marks*

1. Clamp and cut cord.

2. Dry baby and wrap in warm towel.

3. Record 1-minute Apgar score.

4. Rapid inspection for gross abnormalities and birth injuries.

5. Give im vitamin K (if it has been previously discussed and agreed with the mother).

6. Attach label for identification.

7. Hand to mother for early skin-to-skin contact and suckling.

As Alex is born, Debbie is given im oxytocin. After birth, the placenta is removed by controlled cord traction and inspected for completeness.

Give 2 non-pharmacological techniques for reducing postpartum haemorrhage
                                                                   1 mark

Postpartum haemorrhage is caused by failure of uterus to contract (70%), damage to the genital tract (20%), or retained tissue. Uterine contraction, which is under hormonal control of oxytocin, can be increased by:

1. Early suckling, ie stimulates oxytocin release.

2. Rubbing up a uterine contraction, ie massaging the fundus to stimulate a contraction.

Obstetrics & Gynaecology

Name 2 drugs that are used to reduce postpartum haemorrhage   *1 mark*

1. iv Oxytocin (Syntocinon).

2. im Ergometrine.

3. Prostaglandin (F2 alpha-haemobate).

🛈 All these drugs increase uterine contraction.

Total: **20 marks**

4 T's

1° PPH <24h   Tone
(>500ml)   Tissue
                   Trauma
                   Thrombin

2° PPH >24 - 6/52   Infection
                    retained placenta
                    choriocarcinoma.

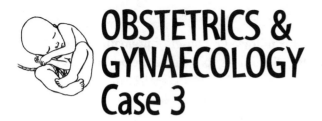

OBSTETRICS & GYNAECOLOGY Case 3

Katie, who is 28 weeks into her first pregnancy, suddenly experiences a gush of fluid vaginally in the absence of any uterine contractions. Cardiotocography (CTG) is normal and ultrasound scan shows residual amniotic fluid. A speculum examination is performed, which reveals a closed cervix and pooling of fluid in the posterior fornix.

List 4 causes of pre-term pre-labour rupture of membranes (PPROM)   *2 marks*

1. Vaginal infection, eg bacterial vaginosis, group B *Streptococcus*.

2. Chorioamnionitis.

3. Cervical incompetence.

4. Antepartum haemorrhage (in particular placental abruption).

5. Urinary tract infection.

6. Multiple gestation.

7. Polyhydramnios.

ⓘ The main causes of PPROM are infection and cervical incompetence.

What common vaginal organism is Katie's baby at risk from?   *1 mark*

1. Group B *Streptococcus*.

ⓘ Group B *Streptococcus* is a commensal organism present in the vagina of up to 25% of women. It may, very rarely, infect the neonate, either during delivery or via ascending infection, eg after PPROM, causing pneumonia, septicaemia or meningitis.

? QUESTIONS
• PAGES 77–80

Obstetrics & Gynaecology

List 2 treatments to minimise perinatal complications **2 marks**

In the majority of cases, PPROM is followed by onset of premature labour. In those cases in which it is not, the dilemma is to balance the advantages of continuing pregnancy so as to increase fetal maturity against the risk of chorioamnionitis (which may cause perinatal death). Both these risks can be minimised by:

1. **Dexamethasone im: should be given to all mothers if < 34 weeks, to promote fetal lung maturity to reduce risk of respiratory distress syndrome.**

2. **Prophylactic antibiotics, ie erythromycin: this may prolong pregnancy and reduce the risk of chorioamnionitis.**

🛈 Tocolytics are contraindicated, as they may prevent delivery in the presence of chorioamnionitis.

On examination, Katie's temperature is 38 °C, her heart rate is 92 bpm and she has increased white cell count and C-reactive protein. In view of the risks of maternal and fetal infection, it is decided to induce labour. Her cervix is assessed using the Bishop's score.

List 4 features used to assess the Bishop's score **2 marks**

Feature	Bishop's score			
	0	1	2	3
Dilatation (cm)	< 1	1–2	2–4	> 4
Length of cervix (cm)	> 4	2–4	1–2	< 1
Station (relative to ischial spines)	- 3	- 2	- 1/0	+ 1/+ 2
Consistency	Firm	Medium	Soft	Soft
Position	Posterior	Middle	Anterior	Anterior

What Bishop's score is considered ripe for induction? **1 mark**

1. A Bishop's score of > 5 indicates that the cervix is favourable for induction.

ⓘ If nulliparous women are induced with an unripe cervix, the risks of prolonged labour, fetal distress and Caesarean section are increased.

What is used to make the cervix ripe for induction?   *1 mark*

1. Intravaginal prostaglandin pessary (or gel).

ⓘ The majority of inductions are started with prostaglandins. Once the cervix is ripe, artificial rupture of the membranes is performed (not relevant in this case); oxytocin infusion may be used to augment contractions.

Katie's contractions are inefficient, so she is started with an infusion of oxytocin.

List 2 potential complications of using oxytocin in Katie   *2 marks*

1. Uterine hyperstimulation: the rate of uterine contraction should be no more than 4 times per 10 minutes; excessive contractions may cause fetal distress. When labour is induced, the fetus requires regular/continuous CTG monitoring.

2. Water intoxication: oxytocin has antidiuretic-hormone-like effects. The risk is reduced by restricting the infusion volume.

ⓘ In a multiparous woman, oxytocin may also cause uterine rupture. When augmenting labour, oxytocin should be used with care as delay may be due to CPD (as opposed to inefficient uterine contractions).

Katie delivers a girl, Jacoba, weighing 1.1 kg. At 1 minute of life, Jacoba's extremities are bluish, her limbs flaccid, her breathing is irregular, she grimaces when the soles of her feet are stimulated and her heart rate is 82 bpm.

Calculate Jacoba's 1-minute Apgar score   *2 marks*

1. 4.

APGAR score			
	0	**1**	**2**
Colour	White/blue	**Extremities blue. Body pink**	Pink
Heart rate	Absent	**< 100**	> 100
Respiratory effort	Absent	**Gasping or irregular**	Regular strong cry
Muscle tone	**Flaccid**	Some flexion of limbs	Active movement
Reflex irritability	Absent	**Grimace**	Cry

Within an hour of birth, Jacoba starts developing signs of respiratory distress. Her trachea is intubated by the neonatologist, artifical surfactant is instilled and her lungs are ventilated by continuous positive airways pressure.

List 4 pulmonary causes of respiratory distress in a neonate   *2 marks*

1. **Transient tachypnoea of the newborn: caused by delay in resorption of lung fluid.**

2. **Respiratory distress syndrome: due to insufficient surfactant production. Affects the majority of neonates born at or before 28 weeks.**

3. **Meconium aspiration.**

4. **Pneumonia, eg group B streptococcal infection is a common cause of neonatal pneumonia (increased risk with PPROM).**

5. **Pneumothorax: occurs spontaneously in up to 1% of deliveries, though often asymptomatic.**

6. **Milk aspiration, eg due to a tracheo-oesophageal fistula, gastro-oesophageal reflux, cleft palate.**

7. **Persistent pulmonary hypertension of the newborn: due to high pulmonary vascular resistance causing right-to-left shunting of blood flow within the heart.**

ⓘ Non-pulmonary causes include congenital heart disease, birth asphyxia and severe anaemia.

Obstetrics & Gynaecology

List 2 complications of artificially ventilating Jacoba's lungs **2 marks**

1. **Retinopathy of prematurity: immature retinal vessels are sensitive to fluctuations in paO_2, causing vascular proliferation leading to retinal detachment and blindness.**

2. **Pulmonary interstitial emphysema: due to air from over-inflated alveoli tracking into the interstitium, reducing lung compliance and worsening respiratory failure.**

3. **Pneumothorax.**

4. **Chronic lung disease of prematurity (bronchopulmonary dysplasia): defined as O_2 requirements past 36 weeks gestational age. Ventilation causes lung damage from pressure trauma, O_2 toxicity and infection.**

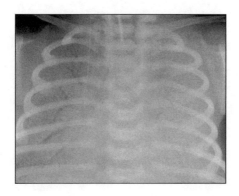

Jacoba's chest X-ray is shown:

Describe 3 abnormalities on the chest X-ray **3 marks**

1. **Endotracheal tube (lies at appropriate position at level of the clavicles).**

2. **Air bronchograms (air in the airways surrounded by solid lung).**

3. **Widespread (or diffuse) shadowing (opacification) of the lungs, often described as ground-glass appearance.**

4. **Indistinct or obscured heart border.**

ⓘ These chest X-ray changes are characteristic of respiratory distress syndrome.

Total: **20 marks**

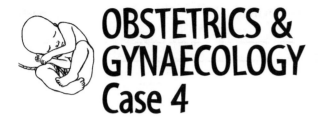

OBSTETRICS & GYNAECOLOGY
Case 4

Paul and Julie (both aged 33 years) visit their GP after 2 years of being unable to conceive. A full history is taken from both. Julie's gynaecological history reveals irregular periods.

List 4 points in a full history suggestive of tubal dysfunction   ***2 marks***

1. Abdominal or pelvic surgery, eg appendectomy.

2. Endometriosis.

3. Peritonitis, eg as a complication of appendicitis.

4. History of pelvic inflammatory disease or sexually transmitted infection.

5. Previous ectopic pregnancy.

6. Tubal ligation (for sterilisation).

🛈 Tubal dysfunction may be due to peritoneal adhesions impairing oocyte pick-up mechanisms (eg in 1–3 above) or impaired tubal patency (eg in 4–6 above).

The GP organises semen analysis for Paul and an outpatient hysterosalpingogram to assess tubal patency in Julie, and requests a number of blood tests.

QUESTIONS
PAGES 81–84

List 4 variables measured in semen analysis   *2 marks*

Variable	Normal range
Volume	> 2 ml
Liquefaction time	Within 60 minutes
Sperm concentration	> 20 million/ml
Total sperm count	> 40 million
Motility	> 50% with normal progression
Morphology	> 30% with normal morphology
WCC	< 1 million/ml

(WCC = white cell count)

🌀If the initial analysis is abnormal, another specimen is evaluated before diagnosis.

The results come back confirming normal semen analysis, and patent tubes. Julie's blood results are shown:

Haemoglobin	12 g/dl (normal range 11.5–16 g/dl)
Rubella	Seronegative
Rhesus	Positive
LH (day 2)	18 units/l (normal range 3–16 units/l)
FSH (day 2)	6 units/l (normal range 2–8 units/l)
Progesterone (day 21)	18 nmol/l (>30)

(LH = luteinising hormone, FSH = follicle-stimulating hormone)

What is a normal day-21 progesterone concentration?   *1 mark*

1. > 30 nmol/l.

Give 2 explanations for Julie's progesterone concentration   *2 marks*

1. Anovulation.

2. Incorrect cycle dates.

🌀 Mid-luteal (day 21) progesterone is measured to confirm ovulation (if it is a 28-day cycle). Progesterone concentration > 30 nmol/l confirms ovulation. If the cycle is irregular, measure 7 days before next suspected period, though this may need to be repeated if the dates are subsequently incorrect.

238

What might a day-2 FSH much greater than 10 units/l suggest?   *1 mark*

1. Premature menopause.

🛈 Significantly increased baseline FSH indicates primary ovarian failure, causing premature menopause (in someone who is aged 33 years).

What is your likely diagnosis?   *1 mark*

1. Polycystic ovarian syndrome (PCOS).

🛈 PCOS is associated with irregular cycles, anovulation, an increased LH producing an LH : FSH ratio ≥ 2 : 1 (normally 1 : 1), and androgen excess. The diagnosis of PCOS is confirmed by ultrasound scan showing multicystic ovaries ('string of pearls' sign, ie peripheral small cysts with increased ovarian volume).

List 3 clinical features which Julie might have   *3 marks*

Typical clinical features of PCOS are:

1. Obesity: approximately 40% of females with PCOS are obese.

2. Acne.

3. Virilisation: development of male secondary sexual characteristics, eg deep voice, clitoromegaly.

4. Hirsutism: presence of excessive facial and bodily hair in a male pattern (though may be disguised)

🛈 PCOS is related to hyperinsulinaemia and insulin resistance causing excessive androgen secretion. Obesity worsens the underlying androgen excess as a result of adipose-tissue conversion of oestrogens to androgens. Treatment of infertility involves weight loss and induction of ovulation with clomiphene (metformin is being increasingly used, though it is not yet licensed for the treatment of PCOS).

Julie is referred to her local infertility clinic, where her infertility is treated with clomiphene.

Obstetrics & Gynaecology

239

List 3 complications associated with this treatment   *3 marks*

1. Ovarian hyperstimulation syndrome: this causes abdominal distension as a result of enlargement of the ovarian cyst and ascites. Complications include thromboembolic events, fluid depletion causing shock, and pulmonary effusions.

2. Multiple pregnancy: affects approximately 20% of clomiphene-treated pregnancies.

3. Ovarian cancer: may increase the risk of ovarian cancer and therefore its use is restricted to 6 months.

List 2 treatments Julie should be offered before conception   *2 marks*

1. Rubella vaccination, as she is seronegative. She would then need to avoid pregnancy within 3 months.

2. Folic acid 0.4 mg/day.

What do IVF-ET, ICSI, GIFT and SUZI stand for?   *2 marks*

1. IVF-ET: **in-vitro fertilisation and embryo transfer.**

2. ICSI: **intracytoplasmic sperm injection.**

3. GIFT: **gamete intrafallopian transfer.**

4. SUZI: **subzonal sperm injection.**

What is the name of the organisation that regulates all assisted conception treatments?   *1 mark*

1. Human Fertilisation and Embryology Authority (HFEA).

Total: *20 marks*

Obstetrics & Gynaecology

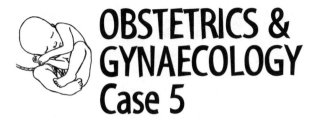

OBSTETRICS & GYNAECOLOGY Case 5

Ageeth, a 26-year-old personal assistant, visits her GP requesting the pill because her new boyfriend doesn't like using condoms.

Describe 3 contraceptive mechanisms of the combined oral contraceptive (COC)

3 marks

1. **Oestrogen and progesterone exert negative feedback on gonadotrophin-releasing hormone, luteinising hormone and follicle-stimulating hormone, preventing follicular development and ovulation.**

2. **Progesterone causes endometrial atrophy, preventing implantation.**

3. **Progesterone acts on cervical mucus, making it hostile to ascending sperm.**

List 6 contraindications to the COC

6 marks

1. **Pregnancy (though there is no evidence that the COC harms the fetus).**

2. **Breast-feeding (as oestrogen inhibits lactation).**

3. **Ischaemic heart disease (IHD) or multiple risk factors for IHD, eg diabetes mellitus, hypertensive, family history.**

4. **Smoker, aged ≥ 35 years and obese (as increased risk of IHD and cerebrovascular accident (CVA)).**

5. **Previous CVA.**

6. **Systemic lupus erythematosus (increased risk of CVA).**

7. **Focal migraine (causes cerebral ischaemia, increasing the risk of CVA).**

Obstetrics & Gynaecology

QUESTIONS
PAGES 85–88

8. Previous deep vein thrombosis/pulmonary embolism (DVT/PE) or **multiple risk factors for DVT, eg thrombophilia, prolonged immobilisation.**

9. Liver disease, eg hepatitis, gallstones.

10. Breast and genital tract cancers (potentially oestrogen sensitive).

🛈 The contraindications to the COC relate mainly to oestrogen inducing a prothrombotic state, increasing the risk of IHD, CVA and DVT/PE. If a COC is contraindicated, the woman may be prescribed the progesterone-only pill (though this is still contraindicated with liver disease, breast and genital tract cancer, IHD and previous ectopic pregnancy).

Nothing in Ageeth's history contraindicates the pill. She is prescribed a 3-month supply of a COC and advised on its side-effects.

Name 6 <u>minor</u> side effects Ageeth may experience   *3 marks*

1. Depression.

2. Headaches.

3. Loss of libido.

4. Nausea and vomiting.

5. Weight gain (due to increased appetite).

6. Bloating/fluid retention.

7. Breast tenderness.

8. Chloasma (facial pigmentation).

9. Spotting (in first few cycles).

10. Oligomenorrhoea.

🛈 More serious (though rare) side-effects include DVT/PE, CVA, IHD, breast and cervical cancer, gallstones and cholestatic jaundice. However, it is worth mentioning the positive side-effects of the COC, including reduced risk of ovarian cancer (and cysts) and endometrial cancer (and uterine fibroids), and reduced pre-menstrual and dysmenorrhoea symptoms.

List 6 pieces of additional advice you would give Ageeth   **3 marks**

1. **When to start the pill, ie start on first day of period, to exclude pregnancy.**

2. **Limitations of the COC, eg doesn't protect against sexually transmitted infections (STIs).**

3. **Factors that reduce its effectiveness, eg: if taking antibiotics, if pill missed > 12 hours, or if diarrhoea and vomiting occur within 3 hours of the pill being taken, alternative contraception must be used for 7 days.**

4. **Availability of emergency contraception.**

5. **Symptoms requiring immediate consultation, eg focal neurological signs, prolonged headache, sudden severe chest pain, shortness of breath, haemoptysis, calf pain, jaundice.**

6. **When you need to see her again, eg repeat prescription, blood pressure check.**

7. **Pre-conception advice, eg take folate supplements, wait for one natural period after stopping pill before attempting conception (to enable accurate dating using last menstrual period).**

Several months later, Ageeth attends her genitourinary medicine clinic complaining of an offensive vaginal discharge.

List 4 additional clinical features that would suggest pelvic inflammatory disease
2 marks

1. **Bilateral lower abdominal pain and tenderness.**

2. **Cervical excitation, ie tenderness when cervix is moved on vaginal examination.**

3. **Adnexal tenderness on vaginal examination.**

4. **Pelvic mass, ie due to a pelvic abscess (woman would be systemically unwell).**

5. **Pyrexia.**

Obstetrics & Gynaecology

243

6. Deep dyspareunia.

7. Menorrhagia.

8. Dysmenorrhoea.

🔟 Pelvic inflammatory disease is typically caused by ascending genital tract infection. Common infective causes include *Chlamydia* and gonorrhoea. Infection may be asymptomatic. Acute symptomatic cases present with vaginal discharge and clinical features 1–5 above; chronic infection may cause vague pelvic pain with additional features 6–8 above. Complications include tubal infertility and ectopic pregnancy.

What 6 questions would you ask in the sexual history?   *3 marks*

1. Number and dates of sexual partners.

2. Whether sex was oral, vaginal and/or anal.

3. What contraception was used.

4. Previous history of STIs.

5. STI history of partner(s), including any current symptoms.

6. Contact details of sexual partners for contact tracing.

7. Human immunodeficiency virus (HIV) status (if known).

8. Hepatitis B virus vaccination status.

List 4 infective causes of vaginal discharge   *2 marks*

1. *Candida albicans* (thrush): infects the vagina. Diagnosed by high vaginal swab (HVS) microscopy (Gram positive) and culture.

2. Bacterial vaginosis (due to abnormal vaginal bacterial flora): infects the vagina. Diagnosed by HVS microscopy, ie clue cells.

3. *Trichomonas vaginalis*: infects the vagina. Diagnosed by HVS microscopy (motile protozoa).

4. *Neisseria gonorrhoeae*: infects the endocervix. Diagnosed by endocervical swab microscopy (Gram negative) and culture.

5. *Chlamydia trachomatis*: infects the endocervix. *Chlamydia* is an intracellular bacterium, so does not Gram stain. Diagnosed by endocervical swab antigen testing.

6. Cervical lesions: syphilis, genital herpes, genital warts. Visualised on speculum examination.

Endocervical and high vaginal swabs are taken. Microscopy reveals pink Gram-stained diplococci.

What is the likely cause of her vaginal discharge? **1 mark**

1. *Neisseria gonorrhoeae*.

Neisseria gonorrhoeae is a Gram-negative diplococcus (and hence stains pink). It primarily infects the endocervical canal in females, causing an offensive vaginal discharge (though it is often asymptomatic; rarely so in males). It may also infect the pharynx (causing pharyngitis) and rectum (causing proctitis) and swabs are also taken from these sites if infection is suspected. Complications include pelvic inflammatory disease and (rarely) disseminated infection causing arthritis and macular rash. It is treated with amoxicillin. Sexual contacts should also be traced and treated.

List 4 additional tests you would offer Ageeth **2 marks**

1. HIV serology. Only positive 3 months after primary infection.

2. Syphilis serology.

3. Hepatitis B virus serology.

4. Cervical smear for cytology if not performed in previous 3 years.

5. Treatment follow-up to confirm eradication of infection.

Total: **25 marks**

PAEDIATRIC CASES:
ANSWERS

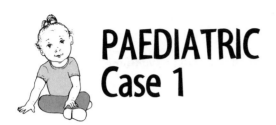

PAEDIATRIC
Case 1

Jim, aged 18 months, is referred to the paediatric outpatient clinic because of poor weight gain over the past 6 months. Apart from two admissions to hospital for bronchiolitis in his first year of life, he was a thriving and happy infant. However, over the past 6 months his mother says he has become irritable, his abdomen seem distended and he has lots of liquid stools, which are foul smelling and difficult to flush. On examination, Jim is pale and his abdomen is protruded. There is wasting of his muscles (especially buttocks) and his ankles seem swollen.

Define failure to thrive **2 marks**

1. Failure to thrive is defined as **poor weight gain (1 mark)** in infants (< 1 year old) and toddlers (1–3 years) with a **fall across 2 or more weight centile lines (1 mark).**

A less strict definition is 'rate of growth that does not meet the expected potential for a child of that age' (score only 1 point). Nowadays, a more parent-friendly alternative term for failure to thrive is 'faltering growth pattern'.

Failure to thrive is demonstrated by plotting sequential weights on the growth chart. A single weight measurement is difficult to interpret unless markedly different from height and head circumference centiles.

List 2 causes for weight below the 0.4th centile other than failure to thrive **2 marks**

1. **Constitutionally small: growth is within predicted range for parental height (this will need to be adjusted for on the growth chart).**

2. **Intrauterine growth retardation.**

QUESTIONS
PAGES 91–93

Paediatric

3. Extreme prematurity.

4. Chromosomal disorders/syndromes, eg Russel-Silver syndrome.

List 3 non-organic causes of failure to thrive   *3 marks*

1. Inadequate food intake, eg because insufficient food offered.

2. Low socioeconomic status, eg unable to afford a good diet.

3. Feeding problems, eg poor breast-feeding technique.

4. Emotional deprivation: results in infant not demanding food (often accompanied by delays in development dependent on stimulation, eg speech).

5. Abuse, eg child neglect; rarely, Munchausen syndrome by proxy, ie mother is deliberately underfeeding child to generate illness.

🛈 Causes of failure to thrive can be classified as organic (underlying pathology) or non-organic (psychosocial and environmental causes). Non-organic causes account for > 95% cases of failure to thrive. Organic causes include gastro-oesophageal reflux disease (poor retention of food), coeliac disease, cystic fibrosis and Crohn's disease (malabsorption), and kidney and heart disease (illness-induced anorexia).

What is the cause of Jim's diarrhoea?   *1 mark*

1. Malabsorption.

🛈 Stools resulting from malabsorption tend to be offensive and difficult to flush down the toilet. Causes of generalised malabsorption can be classified as conditions within the gut lumen (eg cystic fibrosis, bacterial overgrowth) or within the gut mucosa (eg coeliac disease, cow's milk intolerance).

What is the underlying cause of Jim's ankle oedema?   *1 mark*

1. Hypoproteinaemia (hypoalbuminaemia).

🛈 Malabsorption causes intestinal loss of protein, which will lead to a decrease in plasma oncotic pressure. This will cause movement of water from the intravascular to the interstitial space.

As part of his investigations, Jim is screened for cystic fibrosis and coeliac disease.

Briefly outline the cause of diarrhoea in cystic fibrosis and coeliac disease

2 marks

Both cystic fibrosis and coeliac disease cause malabsorption resulting in diarrhoea, though by different underlying mechanisms:

1. Cystic fibrosis: **malabsorption is the result of a deficiency in pancreatic enzymes (amylase, lipase and protease), causing maldigestion with secondary malabsorption.**

2. Coeliac disease: **malabsorption is the result of gluten-provoked mucosal damage in the small bowel, eg villous atrophy, decreasing the area available for absorption.**

List 2 causes of failure to thrive in cystic fibrosis

2 marks

1. **Pancreatic insufficiency: insufficiency of pancreatic enzymes (amylase, lipase and protease) causes malabsorption. This is treated by giving pancreatic enzyme supplements and fat-soluble vitamins.**

2. **Increased energy requirements. Patients with cystic fibrosis have caloric requirements 30–40% greater than normal and are given a high-caloric diet.**

3. **Recurrent chest infections: cause illness-induced anorexia.**

What test do you use to screen for cystic fibrosis and what represents a positive result?

1 mark

1. **Sweat test.**

2. **A positive sweat test for cystic fibrosis is $Na^+ > 60$ mmol/l.**

Paediatric

ⓘ The sweat test is accurate only if more than 100 mg of sweat is collected and chloride is greater than sodium.

Jim's cystic fibrosis screen is negative, but the coeliac disease screen comes back as positive for anti-gliadin and anti-endomysial antibodies. He then undergoes a jejunal biopsy, which histologically confirms coeliac disease.

List 2 jejunal histological changes seen in coeliac disease   *1 mark*

1. Flat jejunal mucosa.

2. Villous atrophy.

3. Lymphocyte infiltration.

How else may coeliac disease present?   *1 mark*

1. Iron- and/or folate-deficient anaemia. This may present with pallor and fatigue (and sometimes pica) with few or no gastrointestinal symptoms.

List 3 food groups Jim will now have to avoid   *3 marks*

Coeliac disease occurs because the proximal small bowel has an inflammatory response to the gliadin fraction in gluten, which is a protein found in:

1. Wheat.

2. Rye.

3. Barley.

Jim is put on a gluten-free diet and within 2 months he has caught up on his growth and is back to his usually happy self. His mother asks whether the diagnosis of coeliac disease is for life.

What do you tell Jim's mother?   *1 mark*

1. **Not necessarily. If coeliac disease presents before 2 years, exclusion of gluten may lead to the jejunum returning to normal. In later childhood, a gluten challenge may be attempted (under medical supervision), after which a biopsy is taken to look for jejunal mucosal damage. If damage is evident, a gluten-free diet should be adhered to for life.**

Total: *20 marks*

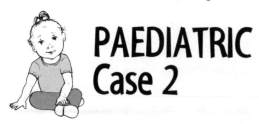

PAEDIATRIC
Case 2

Baby Rebecca is born at 40 weeks gestation, by normal vaginal delivery and weighing 3.2 kg. Her mother (gravida 1, para 1) went into labour spontaneously and labour was not prolonged. Rebecca's Apgar scores were 9 and 10 at 1 and 5 minutes, respectively, and she was transferred to the postnatal ward together with her mother. At the postnatal check the next day, the midwife notices that Rebecca's skin and sclera are yellow. Apart from that she appears very well and is breast-feeding satisfactorily.

Are you concerned about Rebecca's jaundice? Briefly explain your reasoning?

2 marks

1. Yes.

2. Jaundice < 24 hours after birth is always pathological.

ⓘ Jaundice within 24 hours is pathological and may be due to haemolysis or congenital infection. Bilirubin concentrations can increase rapidly and, if unconjugated, (as in haemolysis) may need aggressive treatment. Jaundice after 24 hours may be either pathological or physiological (see below).

Give 3 reasons why jaundice is common in neonates **3 marks**

1. Increased bilirubin production: compared with adults, neonates have a 2- to 3-fold increase in bilirubin production. This is because the haemoglobin concentration decreases rapidly in the first few days after birth, from physiological haemolysis.

2. The half-life of red blood cells is shorter in neonates (70 days) than in adults (120 days).

3. **Immaturity of hepatic bilirubin metabolism: resulting in less efficient bilirubin uptake, conjugation and excretion.**

4. **Breast-feeding: the cause of jaundice in breast-fed infants is unknown.**

Rebecca's jaundice is investigated. Her blood results are shown:

Haemoglobin	12.2 g/dl (normal range 14.5–21.5 g/dl)
Platelets	220 x 10⁹/l (normal range 150–400 x 10⁹/l)
MCV	112 fl (normal range 100–135 fl)
WCC	14 x 10⁹/l (normal range 10–26 x 10⁹/l)
Total serum bilirubin	140 μmol/l (normal range 3–17 μmol/l) (unconjugated)
CRP	< 10 mg/l
Film	Normal RBCs
Rebecca's blood group	A, Rh -ve
Maternal blood group	O, Rh -ve
Direct Coombs' Test	+ (mildly +ve)

(MCV = mean cell volume, WCC = white cell count, CRP = C-reactive protein, RBC = red blood cell, Rh -ve = Rhesus-negative, +ve = positive)

Give 3 causes of increased <u>conjugated</u> bilirubin in neonates $\qquad$ ***3 marks***

1. **Bile duct obstruction.**

2. **Congenital infections, eg TORCH (Toxoplasmosis, Other (e.g. syphilis, HIV) Rubella, CMV, Herpes).**

3. **Neonatal hepatitis.**

🛈 Causes of unconjugated hyperbilirubinaemia include Rhesus and ABO incompatibility, spherocytosis, glucose-6-phosphate dehydrogenase deficiency, neonatal infection (eg urinary tract infection), physiological or breast-milk jaundice and hypothyroidism.

What does the direct Coombs' test detect, and what does it indicate? ***2 marks***

1. **The direct Coombs' test (also called direct antiglobulin test) detects the presence of antibody-coated red blood cells.**

Paediatric

2. This indicates immune-mediated haemolysis, eg Rhesus or ABO incompatibility.

🛈 A positive direct Coombs' test confirms an immune aetiology, though it may be negative in ABO incompatibility.

From the blood results, what is the cause of Rebecca's jaundice?   *2 marks*

1. ABO incompatibility.

🛈 A moderately reduced haemoglobin, increased unconjugated bilirubin and a mildly positive Coombs' test are typically seen in ABO incompatibility. This is confirmed by maternal blood group O and neonatal blood group A. The mother will have circulating anti-A (and anti-B) IgG antibodies, which can cross the placenta and cause immune-mediated haemolysis.

🛈 Rhesus incompatibility is not possible, as both Rebecca and her mother are Rhesus-negative. Blood film is normal, making spherocytosis unlikely (though lack of spherocytes does not totally exclude spherocytosis).

What is your initial management?   *1 mark*

1. Take serial measurements of bilirubin (every 2–4 hours, depending on how steeply concentrations are increasing) and plot on a chart.

🛈 Bilirubin concentrations tend to increase linearly. Therefore, plotting serial concentrations on a chart can be used to predict when phototherapy or exchange transfusion may be required.

Because bilirubin concentrations are increasing (second measurement showed a bilirubin concentration of 280 µmol/l), phototherapy is started.

How does phototherapy work?   *1 mark*

1. Light (blue and white light) converts unconjugated bilirubin by photodegradation into a harmless water-soluble metabolite.

Paediatric

If unconjugated bilirubin reaches high concentrations (> 360 µmol/l) it can become neurotoxic. This happens when bilirubin concentrations exceed the binding capacity of albumin, allowing unbound unconjugated bilirubin to cross the blood–brain barrier.

What is this neurotoxicity called? **1 mark**

1. Kernicterus.

Give 3 signs of this **3 marks**

1. Sleepiness.

2. Poor feeding.

3. Hypotonia.

4. Poor Moro response.

5. High-pitched cry.

6. Arched back (opisthotonus).

Give 2 long-term complications of this **2 marks**

1. Learning difficulties.

2. Cerebral palsy, eg dyskinesia cerebral palsy resulting from deposition of bilirubin in the basal ganglia.

3. Deafness: all babies treated for jaundice undergo hearing tests (brainstem evoked audiometry) before discharge.

Fortunately for Rebecca, phototherapy is successful and she joins her new family at home 4 days later, receiving oral folic acid. She is followed up as an outpatient 2 weeks later for a repeat full blood count, to ensure late haemolysis is not occurring.

Total: **20 marks**

Paediatric

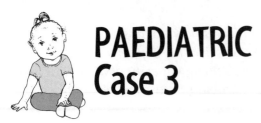

PAEDIATRIC
Case 3

*Erik, aged 8 months, is brought into A&E by his parents 6 days
before Christmas, with a 2-day history of feeding difficulties
preceded by coryzal symptoms. On examination, his temperature is
38.5 °C, he is mildly dehydrated and tachycardic, and has signs of
respiratory distress, with a widespread expiratory wheeze; his saO$_2$
(on air) is 90%.*

List 6 signs of respiratory distress in an infant **3 marks**

1. **Tachypnoea (respiratory rate > 50/min).**

2. **Nasal flaring.**

3. **Subcostal recession.**

4. **Intercostal recession.**

5. **Supracostal recession (tracheal tug).**

6. **Chest hyperinflation.**

7. **Liver displaced inferiorly.**

8. **Cyanosis or pallor.**

9. **Use of accessory muscles, eg causing head bobbing.**

10. **Expiratory grunting: caused by closure of epiglottis in order to try and
    create positive airway pressure during expiration.**

11. **Tachycardia.**

12. **Feeding difficulties.**

QUESTIONS
PAGES 98–100

What are the normal heart rate and respiratory rate in infants?   *2 marks*

Age	Respiratory rate (/min)	Heart rate (bpm)
Infant (< 1 year)	**30–40**	**110–160**
Young child (2–5 years)	20–30	95–140
Older child (5–12 years)	20–25	80–120

List 6 investigations involved in a septic screen   *3 marks*

1. Full blood count: increased white cell count indicates infection.

2. C-reactive protein: may be increased in infection (can be normal in early stages of infection).

3. Blood for microscopy, culture and sensitivities.

4. Chest X-ray: to exclude pneumonia.

5. Urine for microscopy, culture and sensitivities.

6. Lumbar puncture: cerebrospinal fluid for microscopy, culture and sensitivities.

🛈 In febrile infants without an obvious focus for their pyrexia, eg acute otitis media, a septic screen is indicated to exclude severe bacterial infection. In Erik's case, urine analysis and lumbar puncture are not indicated, as the focus of his pyrexia is his lower respiratory tract infection. Additional investigations in Erik would include: **urea and electrolytes: to exclude an electrolyte imbalance, eg syndrome of inappropriate antidiuretic hormone secretion, is a complication of bronchiolitis causing hyponatraemia; nasopharyngeal aspirate: to confirm respiratory syncytial virus (RSV) infection; venous blood gases: to indicate severity of respiratory distress.**

List 4 signs indicating dehydration in an infant   *2 marks*

1. Dry tongue (< 5%).

2. Dull, dry eyes (< 5%).

Paediatric

3. Sunken anterior fontanelle (5–10%).

4. Reduced skin turgor (5–10%).

5. Delayed (ie > 2 s) capillary refill time (5–10%).

6. Irritability (5–10%).

7. Dry nappy, ie oliguria/anuria (> 10%).

8. Weak pulse (> 10%).

9. Reduced blood pressure: normal blood pressure in infant is 90/60 mmHg (> 10%).

🛈 Signs 1–2 above indicate mild dehydration, ie < 5% loss of body weight. Signs 3–6 above (plus earlier signs) indicate moderate dehydration, ie 5–10% loss of body weight. Signs 7–9 above (plus earlier signs) indicate severe dehydration, ie > 10% loss of body weight. This percentage classification is used to calculate fluid replacement requirements.

A diagnosis of bronchiolitis is made and Erik is cohorted on the ward and barrier-nursed to prevent spread of virus.

List 4 types of paediatric patients at risk of bronchiolitis   *2 marks*

1. Prematurity.

2. Chronic lung disease: defined as O₂ therapy beyond 36 weeks of gestation.

3. Congenital heart disease.

4. Down's syndrome.

5. Cystic fibrosis.

6. Immune deficiency, eg severe combined immune deficiency (SCID).

What is the common cause of bronchiolitis and how is it detected?   *2 marks*

1. Respiratory syncytialvirus (RSV): causative agent in approximately 70% of cases (causes winter epidemics).

continues . . .

2. **Nasopharyngeal aspirate for RSV confirmation by immunofluorescent-labelled-antibody detection.**

🛈 Other causes of bronchiolitis include adenovirus, influenza virus and parainfluenza virus.

How would you manage Erik?   *4 marks*

1. **Humidified O_2 by head box or nasal cannulae, with the aim of maintaining $saO_2 > 92\%$.**

2. **Nasogastric feeding. If the infant is unable to tolerate a nasogastric tube, consider iv fluids (5% dextrose + 0.45% saline).**

3. **Antipyretic, eg paracetamol (Calpol). Decreasing the temperature reduces the risk of dehydration and febrile convulsions.**

4. **Continuous saO_2 monitoring: bronchiolitic infants are at risk of apnoea.**

🛈 There is little evidence to support the use of nebulised bronchodilators and steroids. In severe cases, consider nebulised ribavirin (antiviral agent). Antibiotics are not indicated unless secondary bacterial pneumonia is suspected.

How would you monitor the effectiveness of treatment?   *2 marks*

1. **Respiratory rate.**

2. **Heart rate.**

3. **Temperature.**

4. **saO_2.**

5. **Tolerating oral feeds.**

🛈 Discharge criteria are temperature < 38 °C, feeding adequately, saO_2 $> 92\%$ in air, respiratory rate < 50/min and heart rate < 140 bpm.

Total: *20 marks*

Paediatric

261

RESPIRATORY CASES: ANSWERS

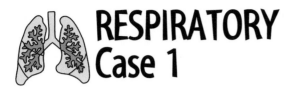

RESPIRATORY
Case 1

Lucy, a 21-year-old asthmatic, presents to A&E with a 2-day history of increased shortness of breath, wheeze and cough. On examination, her temperature is 37.9 °C, her pulse is 125 bpm and her blood pressure 130/80 mmHg; respiratory rate is 30/min, there is widespread bilateral expiratory wheeze and air entry is reduced throughout.

List 3 criteria used to indicate a severe asthma attack   ***3 marks***

1. Can't complete sentences.

2. Respiratory rate > 25/min.

3. Heart rate > 110 bpm.

4. Peak expiratory flow rate (PEFR) < 50% of predicted or best.

List 6 criteria used to indicate a life-threatening asthma attack   ***3 marks***

1. Silent chest.

2. Poor respiratory effort.

3. Exhaustion.

4. Confusion.

5. Cyanosis.

6. Coma.

7. Bradycardia (heart rate < 60 bpm).

8. Hypotension (systolic blood pressure < 90 mmHg).

9. PEFR < 33% of predicted or best.

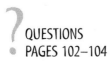

QUESTIONS
PAGES 102–104

Respiratory

10. Respiratory failure ($pO_2 < 8$ kPa).

11. $saO_2 < 92\%$.

What is your immediate management in severe asthma?　　　　　*3 marks*

1. Sit the patient upright and give high-flow (40–60%) O$_2$.

2. Nebulised salbutamol.

3. Hydrocortisone iv/oral prednisolone.

4. Warn the Intensive Therapy Unit (ITU) (if the patient's condition worsens, they may need to be transferred to ITU for tracheal intubation).

What are the 2 indications for iv aminophylline?　　　　　*1 mark*

1. Life-threatening asthma.

2. Poor response to nebulised bronchodilators.

🛈 If the patient is receiving oral theophylline, it is necessary to check that plasma concentrations are within therapeutic ranges. If they are given iv aminophylline, the ECG must be monitored continuously, as there is a risk of fatal arrhythmias (iv salbutamol is a safer alternative).

What 3 brief questions would you ask?　　　　　*3 marks*

1. Ask about usual treatments.

2. Best PEFR: used to assess severity and effect of treatment.

3. Previous admissions to hospital for acute attack, including transfer to ITU (this may give an indication of the potential severity of her asthma).

What 4 blood tests would you do?　　　　　*2 marks*

1. Full blood count: any indication of infection; however, the white cell count is often increased as a result of steroids/stress response.

2. **Urea and electrolytes: any electrolyte imbalance; low potassium associated with the use of ß-agonists.**

3. **C-reactive protein: any indication of infection.**

4. **Arterial blood gases: type I or II respiratory failure.**

5. **Blood cultures: because she is pyrexial.**

ⓘ Also request sputum cultures and sensitivities, to exclude infective exacerbation.

Give 2 reasons why you would request a chest X-ray.   *1 mark*

1. **To exclude a pneumothorax.**

2. **To exclude pneumonia.**

The arterial blood gas results (on air) are shown:

pH   7.31 (normal range 7.35–7.45)

pO_2 7.7 kPa (normal range 10–12 kPa)

pCO_2 3.4 kPa (normal range 4.7–6 kPa)

HCO_3^- 16 mmol/l (normal range 22–28 mmol/l)

What do these results indicate?   *1 mark*

1. **Metabolic acidosis (½ mark) with type I respiratory failure (½ mark).**

ⓘ Normal pH is 7.35–7.45, therefore Lucy's pH of 7.31 is acidotic. It is metabolic acidosis, as opposed to respiratory acidosis, because her pCO_2 is reduced – ie not in keeping with the pH change – and bicarbonate is depleted. This is the result of lactic acid build-up caused by increased respiratory effort. It is type I as opposed to type II respiratory failure, as pO_2 is < 8 kPa but pCO_2 is not increased. The presence of type II respiratory failure is a life-threatening sign requiring tracheal intubation.

Respiratory

267

List 2 ways in which the effects of treatment can be assessed non-invasively

1 mark

1. Clinically, eg respiratory rate, wheeze, ability to complete sentences.

2. Pulse oximetry (SaO$_2$).

3. PEFR.

Lucy's breathing improves and she is transferred to the wards.

What 4 things should Lucy have before discharge?   *2 marks*

1. PEFR > 75% best or predicted and < 20% variability.

2. Inhaler technique checked.

3. Bronchodilator and steroid medications reviewed.

4. Management plan agreed using PEFR monitoring and symptoms.

5. Appointment at respiratory clinic arranged and advised to see GP within 1 week.

Total: *20 marks*

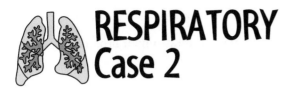

RESPIRATORY
Case 2

Tom, a 73-year-old lifelong smoker with known chronic obstructive pulmonary disease (COPD), is brought into A&E with severe dyspnoea and cough productive of green sputum. On examination, his temperature is 38 °C and his pulse is 95 bpm; his respiratory rate is 35/min, he has widespread expiratory wheeze, reduced air entry throughout and is cyanosed.

List 4 differential diagnoses **2 marks**

1. COPD exacerbation.

2. Pneumonia.

3. Acute pulmonary oedema.

4. Pulmonary embolism.

5. Pneumothorax.

What 4 brief questions would you ask regarding his COPD? **2 marks**

1. Usual treatments including home nebulisers and O$_2$ therapy.

2. Previous acute episodes and their treatment.

3. Normal exercise tolerance.

4. Smoking history.

5. Any allergies to any medications, eg penicillin?

What is your immediate management? **3 marks**

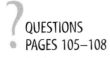

QUESTIONS
PAGES 105–108

Respiratory

1. Controlled O$_2$ therapy (24–28% O$_2$).

2. Nebulised bronchodilators, ie salbutamol and ipratropium bromide.

3. Steroids (iv/oral).

What 4 blood tests would you do? *2 marks*

1. Full blood count: any indication of infection; polycythaemia (due to chronic hypoxia).

2. Urea and electrolytes: any electrolyte imbalance; hypokalaemia from excessive salbutamol use.

3. Arterial blood gases (ABGs): type I or II respiratory failure?

4. C-reactive protein: any indication of infection.

5. Blood cultures: because he is pyrexial.

What 4 non-invasive investigations would you do? *2 marks*

1. Chest X-ray: exclude pneumonia, pulmonary oedema, pneumothorax.

2. ECG: eg may show right heart strain (right axis deviation, dominant R waves in V1, right bundle branch block, peaked P waves); also to exclude co-morbidities.

3. Sputum cultures and sensitivities: identify any infecting organism.

4. Pulse oximetry (saO$_2$).

🛈 Monitoring PEFR in a patient known to have COPD is not recommended, because the magnitude of changes is small compared with the variability of the measurement.

The ABG results (on air) are shown:

pH	7.37 (normal range 7.35–7.45)
pO$_2$	6.9 kPa (normal range 10–12 kPa)
pCO$_2$	4.2 kPa (normal range 4.7–6 kPa)
HCO$_3^-$	25 mmol/l (normal range 22–28 mmol/l)

What do the arterial blood gases indicate? **2 marks**

1. Type I (1 mark) respiratory failure (1 mark).

🛈 pH and bicarbonate are within normal limits. pO_2 is < 8 kPa, ie
respiratory failure, without pCO_2 retention, ie type I as opposed to type II.

How will these results influence your immediate management? **1 mark**

**1. As ABGs do not indicate CO_2 retention, increase to O_2 28–40%, aiming for
$pO_2 > 8$ kPa (need to monitor ABGs regularly).**

List 4 signs of hypercapnia **2 marks**

1. Tachycardia.

2. Bounding pulse.

3. Peripheral vasodilatation.

4. Hand flap.

5. Papilloedema.

6. Confusion.

7. Coma.

🛈 In the presence of type II respiratory failure (ie $pCO_2 > 6$ kPa), O_2 therapy
should be limited to 24–28%, because the respiratory centre is insensitive
to CO_2 and respiration is driven by hypoxia. Excessive O_2 therapy may
cause life-threatening hypercapnia.

*From his past medical history, Tom is considered at high risk of
cardiopulmonary arrest. He informs you of an advance directive
refusing cardiopulmonary resuscitation (CPR).*

List 4 forms in which an advance directive can be made **2 marks**

Advance directives can take several forms:

Respiratory

1. Written document.

2. Witnessed oral statement.

3. A signed card.

4. A note of the discussion in the patient's file.

ⓘ You may also wish to read the following British Medical Association (BMA) paper available at www.bma.org.uk under the ethics section: *Advance statements about medical treatments – code of practice.*

Name 2 of Tom's human rights broken if CPR were to be performed   *2 marks*

1. Article 3: prohibition of torture, inhumane or degrading treatment**: CPR could be considered degrading in that it does not allow a peaceful death.**

2. Article 8: respect for privacy and family life**: Tom has a right to be involved in his medical decisions, including the right to refuse CPR.**

3. Article 9: Freedom of thought, conscience and religion**: Tom has the right of freedom to act upon his beliefs, in this case to refuse CPR.**

4. Article 14: Prohibition of discrimination**: Tom could argue that, by having his advance directive ignored, he is being discriminated against.**

ⓘ You may also wish to read the following BMA paper available at www.bma.org.uk under the ethics section: *The impact of the Human Rights Act 1998 on medical decision making.*

The diagnosis of exacerbation of infective COPD is made; this is successfully treated with amoxicillin.

What 2 organisms are commonly responsible for COPD exacerbations?   *1 mark*

1. *Streptococcus pneumoniae.*

2. *Haemophilus influenzae.*

3. *Moraxella catarrhalis.*

List 4 issues to be addressed on discharge, in collaboration with Tom's GP

2 marks

1. **Smoking cessation.**

2. **Vaccinations: flu (annually) and pneumococcal (ie *Streptococcus pneumoniae* – once only).**

3. **Compliance with regular inhaled treatment.**

4. **Assessment for home O_2.**

List 2 qualifying criteria for home O_2 therapy   *2 marks*

1. **Ex-smoker.**

2. **pO_2 < 7.3 kPa (on 2 separate occasions when COPD is stable at least 3 weeks apart).**

3. **pO_2 < 8 kPa, with evidence of cor pulmonale.**

 The previous criteria of forced expiratory volume in 1 s (FEV1) < 1.5 litre or forced vital capacity (FVC) < 2 litres (on 2 separate occasions when stable at least 3 weeks apart) is not included in the new National Institute for Clinical Excellence (NICE) guidelines. To achieve improved survival, O_2 therapy must be given > 15 hours/day.

Total: *25 marks*

RESPIRATORY
Case 3

Charlotte, a 30-year-old secretary, presents to A&E with sudden onset of severe right-sided chest pain exacerbated by inspiration, with associated breathlessness and feeling dizzy. She is normally fit and well, having recently returned from a week's holiday in Florida with her boyfriend. She is not taking any prescribed medicines except the combined oral contraceptive pill. The abnormal findings on examination are: heart rate 104 bpm, respiratory rate 22/min and a tender, swollen right calf.

List 6 risk factors for pulmonary embolism   ***3 marks***

Risk factors are any cause of immobility or hypercoagulability:

1. **Recent surgery, eg major abdominal or pelvic surgery, hip or knee replacement.**

2. **Prolonged immobilisation, eg plaster cast, bed rest, recent air travel.**

3. **Malignancy, eg abdominal, pelvic, advanced metastatic.**

4. **Pregnancy and puerperium.**

5. **Combined oral contraceptive pill.**

6. **Hormone replacement therapy.**

7. **Hypercoagulability disorders, eg inherited thrombophilia disorders: antiphospholipid syndrome, deficiencies of Factor V Leiden, antithrombin III, protein C or S, thrombin gene mutation.**

8. **Family history of deep vein thrombosis (DVT)/pulmonary embolism.**

9. **Previous DVT/pulmonary embolism.**

Respiratory

QUESTIONS
PAGES 109–111

List 3 differential diagnoses for a tender, swollen calf   **3 marks**

1. Deep vein thrombosis.

2. Cellulitis: erythema suggests cellulitis.

3. Ruptured Baker's cyst.

4. Trauma.

5. Muscle tear.

6. Superficial thrombophlebitis.

🛈 Most pulmonary embolisms arise from venous thrombosis in the pelvis or legs. However, none of the signs of a DVT (eg swollen calf, distended veins, tenderness, increased warmth) is unique to a DVT, which can be reliably confirmed only by Doppler ultrasound examination (if negative but clinical suspicion remains high, use venography or repeat at 10 days).

What is your immediate management?   **2 marks**

1. High-flow O_2

2. Analgesia.

3. Low molecular weight heparin subcutaneously: stop heparin when international normalised ratio (INR) > 2.

4. Start oral warfarin.

5. Antiembolism compression stockings.

6. Stop the pill.

🛈 Thrombolysis is reserved for patients with massive pulmonary embolism causing shock.

What 6 investigations would you do?   **6 marks**

1. Full blood count: polycythaemia, thrombocytosis.

2. Baseline clotting screen: in preparation for anticoagulation.

3. **D-dimer:** a negative D-dimer can accurately exclude a pulmonary embolism. However, it is increased in infection, malignancy and pregnancy in addition to pulmonary embolism, so has a low sensitivity. It is therefore recommended only in excluding pulmonary embolism in patients with low-to-moderate probability of pulmonary embolism (scored in relation to defined clinical criteria).

4. **Chest X-ray:** often normal in pulmonary embolism or small effusion; used to exclude pneumothorax or pneumonia.

5. **ECG:** often normal, though may show sinus tachycardia, right bundle branch block (eg widened QRS complex, RSR [M] pattern in V1), right heart strain (eg dominant R waves in V1–3), right axis deviation (+ve in III, -ve in I); the classical $S_I Q_{III} T_{III}$ (ie deep S waves in I, pathological Q waves and inverted T waves in III) is rare.

6. **Arterial blood gases:** may show reduced pO_2 (with or without reduced pCO_2 as a result of hyperventilation).

7. **Spiral computed tomography scan:** able to detect clots down to the fifth-order pulmonary arteries; or

8. **V/Q scan:** looking for perfusion defects with no corresponding ventilation defects. Reported as low, moderate or high probability of pulmonary embolism, so is interpreted in relation to clinical probability and chest X-ray.

Conventional pulmonary angiogram is no longer routinely used.

Charlotte's ECG is shown:

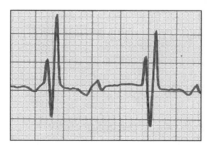

(VI trace shown)

What does this ECG show?   *1 mark*

1. Right bundle branch block (RBBB).

🔵 RSR pattern and widened QRS complex and inverted T wave in V1. May also get deep S wave in V6.

The diagnosis of pulmonary embolism secondary to a DVT is made. Charlotte is discharged on a 6-month course of warfarin with a target international normalised ratio (INR) of 2–3 and an anticoagulant card to carry.

What 4 pieces of general advice would you give to prevent a DVT during a plane flight? **2 marks**

1. Wear compression stockings.

2. Take 75 mg aspirin unless contraindicated.

3. Ensure adequate hydration.

4. Avoid alcohol during the flight.

5. Don't remain seated for long periods – get up and walk around, if only to the toilet.

Six weeks later, Charlotte is treated by her GP with erythromycin (an enzyme inhibitor), for a minor chest infection.

Is she at risk, if so of what and how should this be assessed? **3 marks**

1. Yes: she is at risk, because erythromycin interacts with warfarin; warfarin is metabolised by hepatic cytochrome P450 enzymes, which are inhibited by a number of drugs, including erythromycin.

2. Inhibition of cytochrome P450 will potentiate the anticoagulant effects of warfarin by preventing its metabolism, increasing the risk of haemorrhage.

3. INR should be monitored more closely and the maintenance dose reduced/omitted if target INR is exceeded.

Total: **20 marks**

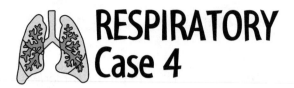

RESPIRATORY
Case 4

Debbie, a 64-year-old heavy smoker, visits her GP complaining of a 3-month history of cough associated with haemoptysis.

List 3 respiratory causes of haemoptysis **3 marks**

1. Acute lower respiratory tract infections.

2. Lung cancer.

3. Tuberculosis.

4. Bronchiectasis: may be a cause of massive haemoptysis.

5. Trauma, eg inhalation of a foreign body.

List 2 other common presenting symptoms of lung cancer **2 marks**

1. Dyspnoea.

2. Chest pain.

3. Anorexia and weight loss.

4. Non-resolving pneumonia.

On examination, the only abnormal finding is that she has clubbing of the fingers.

List 2 cardiac, 2 respiratory and 2 gastrointestinal causes of clubbing **3 marks**

1. Cardiac: **cyanotic congential heart disease, subacute bacterial endocarditis.**

2. Gastrointestinal: **inflammatory bowel disease, cirrhosis, malabsorption (eg coeliac disease), gastrointestinal lymphoma.**

QUESTIONS
PAGES 112–115

3. Respiratory: **lung cancer, chronic lung suppuration (eg cystic fibrosis, bronchiectasis, empyema, abscess), fibrotic lung disease.**

The GP arranges an urgent chest X-ray. The radiological report notes opacification of the right apex, with destruction of the second rib, consistent with bronchial carcinoma.

Debbie's chest X-ray is shown:

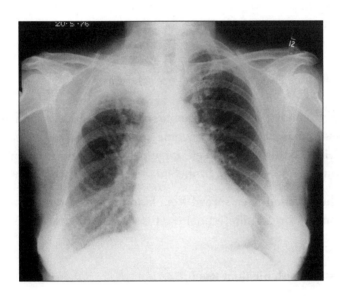

What is this type of lung tumour called?   *1 mark*

1. Pancoast tumour.

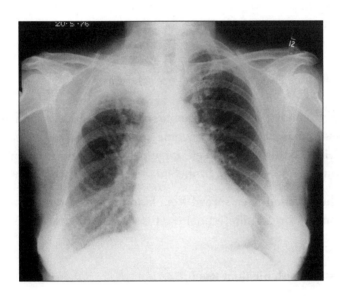 Pancoast tumour refers to a lung tumour in the apex of the lung. It may cause rib erosion, involve the brachial plexus, causing pain down the medial aspect of the arm, or involve the sympathetic chain, causing Horner's syndrome.

List 4 signs of Horner's syndrome   *2 marks*

1. Ptosis: drooping of upper eyelid.

2. Miosis: constricted pupil as a result of unopposed parasympathetic innervation.

3. Enophthalmos: sunken eye.

4. Ipsilateral loss of facial sweating.

ⓘ Lung cancer complications can be classified as local, eg Horner's syndrome, metastatic (spread to liver, bone, brain) and paraneoplastic syndromes (caused by tumour secretory products).

List 4 causes of round lesions on the lung on chest X-ray   *2 marks*

1. Primary lung tumours: most lung tumours are bronchial carcinomas, which can be classified as small-cell carcinoma and non-small-cell carcinoma (further divided into squamous cell, large cell and adenocarcinoma). Rarer forms of lung tumours include bronchiolar-alveolar cell carcinoma.

2. Secondary lung tumours, eg spread from kidney, testis, breast, bone, choriocarcinoma or gastrointestinal tract (usually multiple).

3. 'Round pneumonia'.

4. Abscess (usually with air fluid level).

5. Cyst, eg hydatid.

6. Foreign body.

7. Granuloma (ie nodular accumulation of macrophages), eg tuberculosis, Wegener's syndrome, sarcoid.

8. Arteriovenous malformation (rare).

9. Rheumatoid nodule.

Debbie is seen the following week as an outpatient at the respiratory clinic.

List 3 blood tests you would request **3 marks**

1. Full blood count: may show normocytic anaemia of chronic disease.

2. Liver function tests (LFTs): bronchial carcinoma may metastasise to the liver, causing deranged LFTs.

3. Bone profile: bronchial carcinoma may metastasise to the bones, causing increased Ca^{2+} and increased alkaline phosphatase.

4. Urea and electrolytes: exclude an electrolyte imbalance, eg decreased Na^+ as a result of syndrome of inappropriate antidiuretic hormone secretion (SIADH) (paraneoplastic syndrome).

What 2 investigations would you arrange to confirm lung cancer? **2 marks**

1. Bronchoscopy: to obtain biopsy and washings for histological diagnosis.

2. Chest computed tomography (CT) scan: to stage the tumour.

3. CT-guided biopsy (for peripheral lesions).

🛈 Sputum for cytology is an insensitive test and not routinely performed.

From these tests a diagnosis of inoperable squamous cell bronchial carcinoma is confirmed. Three months later, Debbie is admitted with unremitting back pain causing night-time waking. A lateral spinal X-ray confirms secondary deposits in the thoracic vertebrae. She is treated with radiotherapy and opioid analgesia. The bone profile results are shown:

Ca^{2+} 3.7 mmol/l (normal range 2.12–2.65 mmol/l)

$(PO_4)^{3-}$ 1.4 mmol/l (normal range 0.8–1.45 mmol/l)

ALP   190 iu (normal range 30–150 iu)

$(PO_4)^{3-}$ = phosphate, ALP = alkaline phosphatase

List 5 causes of increased serum calcium **5 marks**

1. Malignant disease: may be caused by bony metastases (common primary tumours are lung, breast, thyroid, prostate, oesophagus, kidney, myeloma) or secretion of parathyroid hormone (PTH)-related protein.

Respiratory

2. **Excessive secretion of PTH:** may be caused by primary or tertiary hyperparathyroidism. Primary is due to parathyroid hyperplasia, adenoma or carcinoma and usually causes mild hypercalcaemia. Secondary is compensatory parathyroid hypertrophy in response to chronic hypocalcaemia (eg in renal failure); calcium concentrations are low or normal. Tertiary is due to prolonged stimulation of the parathyroid in long-standing hypocalcaemia, so that PTH release is no longer under feedback control of calcium.

3. **Hyperthyroidism.**

4. **Excessive calcium intake.**

5. **Excessive vitamin D intake.**

6. **Drugs, eg thiazides (calcium-sparing diuretics).**

7. **Sarcoidosis (producing excess vitamin D).**

🔵 More than 90% of cases of hypercalcaemia are the result of malignancy or hyperparathyroidism.

How would you reduce Debbie's serum calcium? *2 marks*

Acute hypercalcaemia often presents with dehydration as a result of vomiting and polyuria, abdominal pain and constipation and confusion. If the patient is symptomatic or serum Ca^{2+} is > 3.0 mmol/l, reduce hypercalcaemia as follows:

1. **Rehydrate with iv saline (0.9%) 4–6 litres per day: this is to correct any hypovolaemia resulting from vomiting and polyuria.**

2. **Bisphosphonates: inhibit osteoclast activity, thereby reducing bone resorption.**

Total: *25 marks*

RESPIRATORY
Case 5

John, a 63-year-old diabetic carpenter, attends his GP with a 3-day history of cough productive of green sputum, pyrexia and general malaise. He is prescribed amoxicillin, but continues to deteriorate and is admitted to hospital the following day.

John's chest X-ray is shown:

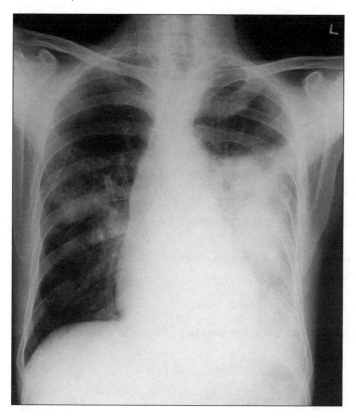

QUESTIONS
PAGES 116–120

283

What is your diagnosis? *1 mark*

1. Left lower lobe pneumonia.

ⓘ Loss of the left hemidiaphragm and preservation of the left heart border indicate that the pneumonia is in the left lower lobe.

List 2 poor prognostic features in the history above *2 marks*

1. 64 years old.

2. Diabetes.

ⓘ Age > 50 years and co-existing chronic disease are associated with a poor prognosis. Failure to respond to treatment would also represent a poor prognostic sign, but in this case John has only received a short course of oral antibiotics. Pyrexia and the production of purulent sputum are not sensitive markers of the severity of pneumonia. Involvement of only one lobe (as opposed to bilateral or multilobar pneumonia) is a good prognostic indicator.

A full examination is performed and blood taken for full blood count, urea and electrolytes, C-reactive protein (CRP), arterial blood gases, liver function tests, glucose and culture.

List 3 findings on <u>examination</u> that would indicate severe pneumonia *3 marks*

1. (New) confusion, ie delirium: eg score of < 9/10 on Abbreviated Mental Test Score (AMTS).

2. Tachypnoea (respiratory rate > 30/min).

3. Hypotension, ie systolic < 90 mmHg or diastolic < 60 mmHg.

List 3 findings on <u>investigation</u> that would indicate severe pneumonia *3 marks*

1. pO_2 < 8 kPa (or saO_2 < 92%), regardless of inspired oxygen concentration.

2. Increased urea (> 7 mmol/l).

3. White cell count > 20 x 10^9/l (leucocytosis) or < 4 x 10^9/l (leucopenia).

4. Positive blood culture.

ⓘ Bilateral or multilobe pneumonia on chest X-ray would also indicate severe pneumonia (though not relevant in this case).

ⓘ The British Thoracic Society CURB-65 score is a simple tool for assessing severity, judging that presence of 3 or more of the following indicates severe pneumonia (which is treated with iv cephalosporin + macrolide): **c**onfusion < 9/10 AMTS; **u**rea > 7 mmol/l ; **r**espiratory rate > 30/min; **b**lood pressure, systolic < 90 mmHg or diastolic < 60 mmHg age > 65 years.

John is treated with O_2 to maintain his arterial oxygen saturation $(saO_2) > 92\%$, paracetamol for his pleuritic chest pain and oral antibiotics (amoxicillin and erythromycin, to cover atypical organisms).

List 3 causes of 'atypical' pneumonia   *3 marks*

1. *Mycoplasma pneumoniae.*

2. *Legionella pneumophila.*

3. *Coxiella burnetii* (Q fever): infection is acquired from animals, eg sheep.

4. *Chlamydia* spp., eg *Chlamydia psittaci, Chlamydia pneumoniae.*

ⓘ Mycoplasma infection occurs in epidemics approximately every 4 years. In a non-epidemic year, atypical organisms account for only 3% of cases. Atypical infections do not respond to penicillin, and require macrolides or quinolones.

List 6 parameters used to assess the progress of treatment   *3 marks*

1. Heart rate.

2. Respiratory rate.

3. Blood pressure.

4. Temperature.

5. saO_2 (or O_2 requirements necessary to maintain adequate saO_2).

6. Mental status.

Respiratory

7. CRP: this is a sensitive marker of treatment progress.

8. White cell count.

🄳 In patients not progressing satisfactorily, the chest X-ray should be repeated to look for complications.

John's blood results are shown:

Hb	13.1 g/dl	CRP	267 mg/l	pH	7.39
MCV	85 fl			pO_2	9.1 kPa
Platelets	320 x 10⁹/l	Glucose	8.2 mmol/l	pCO_2	4.9 kPa
WCC	14 x 10⁹/l			HCO_3^-	24 mmol/l
		Bilirubin	11 µmol/l		
Na⁺	141 mmol/l	ALT	17 iu/l	Blood culture	Gram +ve cocci
K⁺	4.6 mmol/l	AST	14 iu/l		
Urea	6.1 mmol/l	ALP	54 iu/l		
Creatinine	112 mmol/l				

(Hb = haemoglobin, MCV = mean cell volume, WCC = white cell count, CRP = C-reactive protein, ALT = alanine aminotransferase, AST = aspartate aminotransferase, ALP = alkaline phosphatase, pO_2, pCO_2 = partial pressures of oxygen and carbon dioxide, HCO_3^- = bicarbonate)

What is the most likely cause of John's pneumonia, and how can this be prevented?   *2 marks*

1. *Streptococcus pneumoniae* is a **Gram-positive (ie stains purple) coccus and is the most common cause of pneumonia (*Staphylococcus* is also a Gram-positive coccus, but is not a common cause of commonly acquired pneumonia).**

2. **Pneumococcal vaccination: should be offered to all those with a chronic illness, eg diabetes mellitus.**

John's temperature and CRP remain high and clinical examination reveals reduced breath sounds at the right base. His chest X-ray is repeated (and shows a right pleural effusion).

What is the most likely complication? **1 mark**

1. Empyema.

ⓘ Empyema refers to pus in the pleural space. The fluid should be tapped and sent for pH analysis. If the pH is < 7.2, the effusion should be treated as an empyema. Other complications of pneumonia that may be seen on chest X-ray include pleural effusion and lung abscess (cavitating area of localised suppurative (pus forming) infection).

How should this be treated? **2 marks**

1. Tube drainage. Intrapleural fibrinolytic, eg streptokinase, is given twice daily into the drain to liquefy pus and aid drainage.

2. High dose intravenous antibiotics.

Total: **20 marks**

RHEUMATOLOGY CASES: ANSWERS

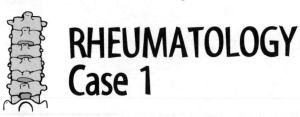

RHEUMATOLOGY
Case 1

Kristine, a 36-year-old nurse, is referred to the Rheumatology outpatient department with a 2-month history of stiff, painful, swollen hands associated with general malaise.

List 4 inflammatory causes of polyarthropathy   **4 marks**

1. **Rheumatoid arthritis (RA): systemic disease causing a symmetric polyarthritis.**

2. **Reactive arthritis: arthritis following infection, eg post-dysentery or non-gonococcal urethritis (ie Reiter's syndrome).**

3. **Viral arthritis, eg hepatitis B virus or mumps.**

4. **Connective tissue disorders, eg systemic lupus erythematosus (SLE).**

5. **Seronegative arthritides, eg associated with psoriasis, ankylosing spondylitis and inflammatory bowel disease.**

6. **Lyme disease: tick-borne infection caused by *Borrelia burgdorferi*.**

7. **Polymyalgia rheumatica: typically affects older women, causing myalgia, stiffness and polyarthritis.**

Examination of Kristine's hands and wrists shows changes characteristic of rheumatoid arthritis (RA).

Give 8 features of RA in the hands and wrists on examination   **4 marks**

1. **Boggy swelling (synovitis) of small joints of hands (metacarpophalangeal (MCP), proximal interphalangeal (PIP) and distal interphalangeal (DIP) joints).**

2. **Tender, erythematous, hot joints.**

QUESTIONS
PAGES 122–124

3. Loss of valleys around the knuckles on making a fist: due to MCP joint swelling.

4. Sausage shaped fingers (spindling): due to soft-tissue swelling.

5. Wasting of intrinsic muscles of the hand.

6. Swan-neck deformity: fixed hyperextension of PIP joint and flexion of DIP joint.

7. Boutonniere (or button-hole) deformity: fixed flexion of PIP joint.

8. Z-deformity of the thumb.

9. Finger drop: due to rupture of finger extensor tendons (following wrist subluxation).

10. Subluxation of the wrist.

11. Prominent radial head (piano key).

12. Loss of function.

13. Symmetric changes, ie involvement of both hands.

ⓘ RA typically presents slowly, evolving over weeks to months with stiff, painful, swollen hands and feet, before progressing to involve larger joints, eg shoulders, knees.

Kristine is sent for an X-ray of her hands.

Give 4 X-ray changes in the hands in RA   *2 marks*

Early changes:

1. Soft-tissue swelling.

2. Juxta-articular osteoporosis.

3. Loss of joint space.

Late changes:

1. Bony erosions at the joint margins.

2. Subluxation and dislocation of joints.

3. Carpal bone destruction.

🛈 Other investigations include: full blood count (normochromic anaemia, increased white cell count), erythrocyte sedimentation rate (ESR) and/or C-reactive protein (CRP), rheumatoid factor (RF) and anti-nuclear antibody (positive in 30% of patients).

🛈 RFs are autoantibodies directed at antibodies, eg anti-IgG IgM. Although often negative at the start of RA, they are eventually positive in 70–80% of patients. However, RFs are not diagnostic of RA (though they are prognostic), also occurring in connective tissue disorders such as SLE. The term 'seronegative RA' (and other seronegative arthritides) refers to patients without RFs and in whom the joint involvement tends to be more limited.

List 4 criteria on history, examination and investigation used to diagnose RA in Kristine **4 marks**

1. **Morning stiffness > 1 hour.**

2. **Arthritis of ≥ 3 joints.**

   For ≥ 6 weeks

3. **Arthritis of hand and wrist joints.**

4. **Symmetric arthritis.**

5. **Rheumatoid nodules (most common at sites of pressure, eg extensor surfaces of forearm).**

6. **Rheumatoid factor seropositive.**

7. **Typical radiological changes.**

🛈 RA is diagnosed on the basis of 4 or more positive criteria.

List 4 features associated with a poor prognosis **2 marks**

1. **Female sex.**

2. **Multiple joint involvement.**

3. **Early functional disability.**

4. **Early X-ray changes.**

5. **Extra-articular features.**

6. **Persistently high CRP/ESR.**

7. **Human leukocyte antigen (HLA) DR4-positive.**

8. **High titres of RF.**

🌑 RA is a systemic disease affecting many organs: eyes (Sjögren's syndrome (dry eyes), scleritis, scleromalacia perforans), cardiovascular system (pericarditis, pericardial effusions, Raynaud's disease), respiratory system (pleural effusions, nodules and Caplan's syndrome; fibrosing alveolitis, bronchiectasis), skin (ulcers, nodules, vasculitis, pyoderma granulosum), nervous system (carpal tunnel syndrome, peripheral neuropathy, mononeuritis multiplex, cervical myelopathy), Felty's syndrome (splenomegaly and neutropenia that are associated with infections, anaemia, thrombocytopenia and lymphadenopathy), kidneys (renal failure).

Kristine is diagnosed with RA and initially treated with non-steroidal anti-inflammatory drugs. However, because of pain and progressive loss of function, her rheumatologist prescribes a disease-modifying antirheumatic drug (DMARD).

Name 2 DMARDs and 2 side-effects associated with each   *4 marks*

DMARD		Associated side-effects
1.	Methotrexate	Hepatotoxicity, bone-marrow suppression, pulmonary toxicity, mucositis (eg mouth ulcers)
2.	Sulphasalazine	Bone-marrow suppression, oligospermia, skin rash, GI intolerance (eg nausea), hepatotoxicity
3.	Penicillamine	Skin rash, proteinuria (may progress to renal failure), GI intolerance (metallic taste, nausea)
4.	Gold	Proteinuria (may progress to renal failure), skin rash, blood dyscrasia, GI intolerance (eg diarrhoea)
5.	Antimalarials, ie hydroxychloroquine and chloroquine	Corneal deposits, retinopathy
6.	Azathioprine	Bone-marrow suppression, hepatotoxicity, GI intolerance (eg nausea)
7.	Cyclophosphamide	Bone-marrow suppression, carcinogenesis, pulmonary toxicity, GI intolerance (eg nausea), cardiac toxicity (eg heart failure, arrhythmias)
8.	TNF inhibitors, ie infliximab, etanercept	Infections (eg TB, septicaemia), worsening heart failure, injection-site reactions and blood dyscrasias

(DMARD = disease-modifying antirheumatic drug; GI = gastrointestinal; TNF = tumour necrosis factor alpha; TB = tuberculosis)

Rheumatolog

🛈 Treatment of RA includes patient education, physical therapy, splints, surgery and pharmacological treatments. Pharmacological treatments include simple analgesia, non-steroidal anti-inflammatory drugs (NSAIDs), corticosteroids (both orally and by intra-articular injection; used for acute exacerbations and to control symptoms while DMARDs are being introduced) and DMARDs, including the newer biological agents, eg tumour necrosis factor alpha (TNF alpha) inhibitors.

🛈 DMARDs suppress the disease process in RA (as indicated by reductions in symptoms and joint swelling, decrease in ESR/CRP and retardation in radiological joint damage), typically through inhibition of cytokines; unlike NSAIDs, however, they take several months to achieve a full response. They are typically prescribed in patients with poor prognostic features (see above). Patients are initially prescribed either methotrexate or sulphasalazine; those with a poor response to initial therapy are changed to an alternative DMARD, or are commenced on combination DMARD therapy (recently it has been shown that methotrexate and TNF alpha inhibitors act synergistically in combination).

🛈 TNF alpha inhibitors have been recommended by the National Institute for Clinical Excellence for the treatment of highly active RA when the patient has failed to respond to 2 DMARDs. Prescribing and monitoring of these agents should be undertaken by a rheumatologist, and they should be withdrawn after 3 months if there is no response to treatment or if serious side-effects develop. They are very expensive.

Total: 20 marks

UROLOGICAL CASES:
ANSWERS

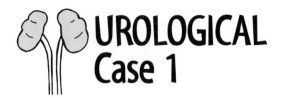

UROLOGICAL
Case 1

Rommy, a 49-year-old busy housewife, is investigated for malaise and fatigue by her GP. Her current medications are insulin, angiotensin converting enzyme inhibitor (ACEI; for hypertension) and non-steroidal anti-inflammatory drug (NSAID; for chronic back pain). Her blood results are shown:

Hb	9.2 g/dl	Na$^+$	136 mmol/l
MCV	86 fl	K$^+$	5.7 mmol/l
WCC	5.2 x 10^9/l	Urea	27 mmol/l
Platelets	280 x 10^9/l	Creatinine	195 µmol/l
Glucose	18.7 mmol/l	Ca^{2+}	1.82 mmol/l
HbA1c	9.2%	(PO$_4$)$^{3-}$	2.72 mmol/l

(Hb = haemoglobin, MCV = mean cell volume, WCC = white cell count, HbA1c = glycated haemoglobin, (PO$_4$)$^{3-}$ = phosphate)

List 3 blood tests suggestive of chronic renal failure **3 marks**

Rommy has renal failure as indicated by her increased urea (2.5–6.7 mmol/l) and creatinine (70–150 µmol/l). The following blood tests suggest chronic, as opposed to acute, renal failure:

1. Normochromic normocytic anaemia: haemoglobin < 11.5 g/dl.

2. Hypocalcaemia: reduced calcium (2.12–2.65 mmol/l).

3. Hyperphosphataemia: increased phosphate (0.8–1.45 mmol/l).

ⓘ Previous abnormal urea and electrolytes and small kidneys on ultrasound scan also suggest chronic renal failure.

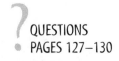

QUESTIONS
PAGES 127–130

What is the likely cause of her anaemia? *1 mark*

1. Erythropoietin (EPO) deficiency.

🔘 The kidneys release EPO to stimulate erythropoiesis in the bone marrow. Chronic renal failure causes a deficiency in EPO, resulting in anaemia. This is corrected by excluding other causes (eg iron and folate deficiency) and giving EPO. Blood transfusion should be avoided as it increases the risk of human leukocyte antigen (HLA) sensitisation and hence tissue rejection in renal transplantation.

Name 4 factors that might be contributing to Rommy's renal failure *2 marks*

1. Poorly controlled diabetes mellitus (as indicated by HbA1c > 7%): causing diabetic nephropathy.

2. Hypertension: causing hypertensive nephropathy.

3. ACEI: may cause acute renal failure as a result of reduced renal perfusion in patients with renal artery stenosis.

4. NSAID: may cause tubulointerstitial nephritis, leading to renal failure.

🔘 Complications of hypertension and diabetes mellitus include renal failure, the risk of which is reduced by tight control. ACEIs have been shown to reduce the rate of progression of renal failure in patients with diabetes.

List 4 <u>systemic</u> causes of pruritus *2 marks*

The causes of pruritus can be classified as local (eg eczema, infestation) and systemic:

1. Chronic renal failure (uraemia).

2. Jaundice (due to bile salts).

3. Polycythaemia rubra vera.

4. Iron-deficient anaemia.

5. Hypothyroidism.

6. Cancer, eg lymphoma (B symptoms).

7. Drugs, eg combined oral contraceptive, morphine.

🛈 Chronic renal failure may cause a range of symptoms, including malaise, lethargy, nocturia and polyuria, pruritus, bone pain, nausea and vomiting, restless leg syndrome and symptoms of anaemia.

Rommy is referred to a nephrologist for her chronic renal failure and is kept under review for progression of her disease and to prevent or treat any complications.

List 2 treatments to prevent renal bone disease   *2 marks*

Renal bone disease is prevented by aggressively treating hypocalcaemia and hyperphosphataemia, by:

1. Dietary phosphate restriction, eg less milk, cheese, eggs.

2. Phosphate binders: use of calcium-containing phosphate binders is often limited by causing hypercalcaemia; newer treatments, including sevelamer, cause fewer side-effects.

3. Alphacalcidol or calcitriol to correct 'activated' vitamin D deficiency.

🛈 Renal bone disease is caused by reduced renal phosphate excretion resulting in hyperphosphataemia, which in turn stimulates the release of parathyroid hormone (PTH). There is also reduced vitamin D activation, resulting in reduced dietary Ca^{2+} absorption (causing hypocalcaemia) and increased PTH release. PTH acts to promote bone Ca^{2+} resorption (also causes resorption of $(PO_4)^{3-}$), in addition to promoting renal Ca^{2+} reabsorption (and renal $(PO_4)^{3-}$ excretion) to oppose any hypocalcaemia, ultimately causing bone disease.

How would you monitor the effectiveness of such treatment?   *1 mark*

1. Monitor PTH concentrations.

🛈 PTH is measured regularly to assess whether hyperparathyroidism is being effectively suppressed by treating hypocalcaemia and hyperphosphataemia.

Urological

A graph of Rommy's reciprocal plasma creatinine concentration against time is shown:

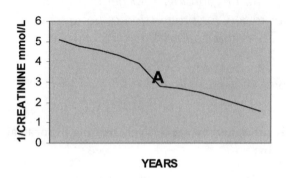

RENAL FUNCTION

Give 4 possible causes for the sharp decline at time A   **2 marks**

Renal function is monitored by reciprocal plots of plasma creatinine. Normally, the decline is linear, so any rapid decline needs investigating to slow down the ultimate progression to end-stage renal failure and dialysis. Causes of rapid decline include:

1. Uncontrolled hypertension.

2. Uncontrolled diabetes mellitus.

3. Infection.

4. Dehydration.

5. Nephrotoxic drugs, eg NSAIDs.

6. Urinary tract obstruction.

7. Hypercalcaemia.

Rommy is referred for haemodialysis when her plasma creatinine reaches 650 µmol/l and is put on the waiting list for renal transplantation.

List 3 other indications for dialysis in chronic renal failure   *3 marks*

1. **Hyperkalaemia, ie K$^+$ > 6.5 mmol/l: prevent by reducing dietary potassium, eg bananas; avoid potassium-sparing diuretics.**

2. **Severe metabolic acidosis, ie pH < 7.2; HCO$_3^-$ < 15 mmol/l: treat by giving sodium bicarbonate supplements.**

3. **Severe uraemic symptoms: eg confusion (which is prevented by reducing dietary protein), neuropathy, nausea and vomiting.**

4. **Refractory pulmonary oedema: prevent by reducing sodium and fluid intake.**

5. **Pericarditis.**

6. **Poor control of renal function by conservative treatment.**

7. **Accelerated hypertension, poorly responsive to antihypertensive medication.**

Give 2 arguments for and 2 arguments against commercial kidney donation
4 marks

For:

1. **Selling a kidney promotes the autonomy of the vendor, ie their right to sell their own kidney.**

2. **Opportunity to buy a kidney promotes the autonomy of the recipient, ie increases the options for a patient in end-stage renal failure.**

3. **Helps reduce the kidney transplant waiting list.**

4. **Commercial kidney donation already exists on the black market. Its legalisation would prevent its abuse and safeguard both vendors and recipients.**

Against:

1. **May lead to exploitation of vulnerable individuals.**

2. **Discriminates against poor people, ie only wealthy patients will be able to afford a transplant.**

3. **Selling kidneys may result in the slippery slope of selling other vital organs, eg hearts.**

Urological

4. Selling kidneys will reduce the public's confidence in the medical profession because of its association with a money-making practice.

ⓘ You may also wish to read the following paper available at www.thelancet.com: Radcliffe-Richards *et al*. The case for allowing kidney sales. *Lancet* 1998; 352: 1950–1952.

Total: *20 marks*

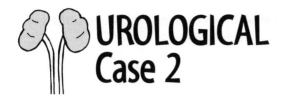

UROLOGICAL
Case 2

Friso, a 39-year-old managing director, presents to A&E with severe left-sided loin pain radiating down to his groin; he also complains of vomiting and sweating.

List 3 urine chemical abnormalities predisposing to urinary stone formation

3 marks

1. Hypercalciuria.

2. Hyperuricosuria.

3. Hyperoxaluria.

4. Cystinuria.

There are various types of urinary stones: calcium oxalate, calcium phosphate, magnesium ammonium phosphate, uric acid and cystine stones. Risk factors include chemical composition in blood or urine favouring stone formation, dehydration, pyelonephritis and kidney disease.

List 2 findings on urine dipstick suggestive of a urinary tract infection   *1 mark*

Complications of urinary stone disease include urinary tract infection and obstructive uropathy, which may cause hydronephrosis. Infective hydronephrosis is termed pyonephrosis and all patients presenting with pyelonephritis must undergo a renal ultrasound scan to exclude pyonephrosis, which is treated by emergency nephrostomy.

1. Nitrites: Gram-negative bacteria (eg *Escherichia coli*) reduce nitrates to nitrites.

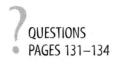

QUESTIONS
PAGES 131–134

Urological

2. **Leukocytes: measures esterase released by leukocytes. Pyuria (ie white cells in the urine), is defined as > 10 white cells/mm^3.**

3. **Haematuria.**

ⓘ Mid-stream urine should also be sent for microscopy, culture and sensitivities. Growth > 10^5 colony-forming units/ml is considered diagnostic of a urinary tract infection.

Name 2 bacterial causes of urinary tract infection   *1 mark*

1. *Escherichia coli*: **most common cause.**

2. *Proteus mirabilis.*

3. *Klebsiella aerogenes.*

4. *Enterococcus faecalis.*

5. *Staphylococcus saprophyticus*: **common in sexually active young females.**

6. *Staphylococcus epidermidis.*

7. *Pseudomonas aeruginosa.*

8. *Serratia marcescens.*

ⓘ The last 3 organisms are more commonly found in hospital-acquired urinary tract infections, eg from catheters. *Mycobacterium tuberculosis* causes sterile pyuria. Culture early morning urines specifically for mycobacteria if this is a possible diagnosis.

ⓘ Lower urinary tract infections (ie cystitis, causing frequency, urgency, dysuria, suprapubic pain and haematuria) are treated with trimethoprim or co-amoxiclav. Upper urinary tract infections (ie pyelonephritis, additionally causing loin pain, rigors and fever) are treated with more prolonged courses of antibiotics and may require iv cephalosporins or ciprofloxacin.

Friso's film is shown, demonstrating a dilated left renal pelvis, clubbed calyces and ureteric obstruction:

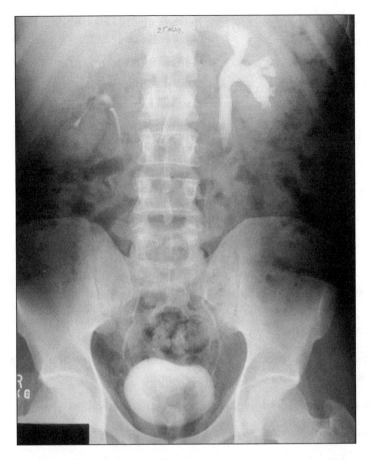

What is the name of this investigation? **1 mark**

1. Intravenous urography.

Intravenous urography involves serial, timed abdominal X-rays after iv injection of a contrast medium. It may show a filling defect, failure of contrast to pass distally beyond a ureteric stone, dilatation of the proximal urinary tract, or impaired renal function (weak and/or delayed excretion of contrast).

Other basic investigations in urinary stone disease include abdominal X-ray (80% of urinary stones are radio-opaque), full blood count (any indication of infection), urea and electrolytes (any indication of renal impairment), mid-stream urine for microscopy, culture and sensitivities (exclude infection). Ultrasound is also used to demonstrate structural abnormalities.

Urological

305

Friso's urea and electrolyte data indicate acute renal failure with hyperkalaemia.

List 2 causes each of pre-renal, renal-renal and post-renal failure   **6 marks**

Pre-renal failure is caused by renal hypoperfusion:

1. Any cause of hypovolaemia, eg haemorrhage.

2. Sepsis.

3. Decreased cardiac output, eg heart failure, cardiac tamponade.

4. Renal artery stenosis.

5. Drugs, ie non-steroidal anti-inflammatory drugs (NSAIDs) and angiotensin converting enzyme inhibitors (ACEIs) decrease renal blood flow.

Renal-renal failure may be caused by:

1. Acute tubular necrosis: this is the most common cause of acute renal failure and is typically caused by renal ischaemia.

2. Acute tubulointerstitial nephritis, eg NSAIDs, penicillin.

3. Pyelonephritis.

4. Glomerulonephritis: immune-complex-mediated damage to the glomerulus, eg systemic lupus erythematosus.

5. Hepatorenal syndrome

Post-renal failure is caused by obstruction to the renal tract anywhere from the calyces to the external urethral orifice:

1. Urinary stone disease.

2. Benign prostatic hypertrophy.

3. Prostatic carcinoma.

4. Pelvic or abdominal tumours.

5. Retroperitoneal fibrosis, eg methyldopa, ß-blockers.

List 4 causes of hyperkalaemia   *2 marks*

Hyperkalaemia is caused by either increased cellular release of potassium or failure of its excretion. Increased cellular release may occur in:

1. **Metabolic acidosis, eg diabetic ketoacidosis: due to cellular exchange of K+ for H+.**

2. **Cell lysis, eg rhabdomyolysis, blood transfusion.**

3. **Digoxin toxicity: due to inhibition of Na+/K+ pump.**

4. **Artefactual: haemolysis of blood sample.**

Failure of excretion may occur in:

1. **Renal failure: both acute and chronic renal failure.**

2. **Potassium-sparing diuretics, eg spironolactone.**

3. **ACEIs: inhibit aldosterone-mediated K+ excretion.**

4. **Addison's disease, ie aldosterone deficiency.**

5. **Acidosis: H+ competes with K+ for excretion in the distal convoluted tubule.**

Give 2 ECG changes associated with hyperkalaemia   *1 mark*

1. **Tall-tented T waves.**

2. **Small P waves.**

3. **Increased PR interval.**

4. **Widened QRS complex.**

ⓘ Hyperkalaemia causes hyperpolarisation of cell membranes, leading to reduced cardiac excitability predisposing to arrhythmias. It requires emergency treatment if > 6.5 mmol/l or associated with the above ECG changes.

How would you treat life-threatening hyperkalaemia?   *3 marks*

Urological

1. **Calcium gluconate iv (if ECG changes present): cardioprotective, though does not reduce serum potassium concentrations.**

2. **Glucose and insulin iv: insulin promotes cellular uptake of K+ (glucose to counteract the effects of insulin); nebulised ß-agonists also drive potassium into cells.**

3. **Bicarbonate iv if severe metabolic acidosis.**

4. **Calcium resonium (oral or rectal): the only treatment that actually removes potassium from the body.**

ⓘ If refractory hyperkalaemia, consider dialysis.

Friso's hyperkalaemia does not warrant urgent treatment. He undergoes nephrostomy to relieve his upper urinary tract obstruction and his ureteric stone is successfully fragmented by extracorporeal shockwave lithotripsy (ESWL). His urea and electrolyte data subsequently indicate recovery of his renal function.

Name 2 early complications following recovery from acute renal failure *2 marks*

In the early stages of acute renal failure, recovery may reach a diuretic phase in which glomerular filtration rate > renal reabsorption, causing:

1. **Hyponatraemia.**

2. **Hypokalaemia**

3. **Hypovolaemia.**

Total: *20 marks*

Urological

INDEX

*This index covers the answer section only. Page numbers in **bold** indicate the main subject of each case.*

REFERENCES

The core references that we have used in writing this textbook are shown below and are probably books you already own (or at least have access to). However, we have also used, where available, published national or local guidelines to ensure that all the information in this textbook reflects best current practice; these national guidelines are freely available on the internet following the hyperlinks given (the local guidelines will be available in your hospital).

CORE REFERENCES

Campbell S, Lees C. Obstetrics by Ten Teachers: 17th Edition. 2000. Arnold. ISBN: 0-340-71986-9.

Campbell S, Monga A. Gynaecology by Ten Teachers: 17th Edition. 2000. Arnold. ISBN: 0-340-71987-7.

Collier J, Longmore M, Duncan-Brown T. Oxford Handbook of Clinical Specialties: 5th edition. 1999. Oxford University Press. ISBN: 0-19-262943-3.

Kumar P, Clark M. Clinical Medicine: 4th Edition. 1999. WB Saunders. ISBN: 0-7020-2019-2.

Lissauer T, Clayden G. Illustrated Textbook of Paediatrics: 2nd Edition. 2001. Mosby. ISBN: 0-7234-3178-7.

Longmore M, Wilkinson I, Torok E. Oxford Handbook of Clinical Medicine: 5th Edition. 2001. Oxford University Press. ISBN: 0-19-262988-3.

PUBLISHED GUIDELINES

CARDIOLOGY CORE CASES

Heart Failure
Chronic heart failure: Management of chronic heart failure in adults in primary and secondary care: National Institue of Clinical Excellence (NICE) guideline.
http://www.nice.org.uk

Angina
Management of stable angina: Scottish Intercollegiate Guidelines Network (SIGN) guideline.
http://www.sign.ac.uk

Hypertension
Williams B. et al. British Hypertension Society guidelines for hypertension management 2004 (BHS-IV): summary. BMJ, 2004; 328: 634 - 640.
http://www.bmj.com

Myocardial Infarction
National Service Framework for Coronary Heart Disease.
http://www.dh.gov.uk

GASTROENTEROLOGY CORE CASES

Dyspepsia
British Society of Gastroenterology (BSG) dyspepsia management guidelines.
http://www.bsg.org.uk

Pancreatitis
United Kingdom guidelines for the management of acute pancreatitis: BSG guideline.
http://www.bsg.org.uk

Inflammatory bowel disease
Inflammatory bowel disease: BSG management guidelines.
http://www.bsg.org.uk

NEUROLOGICAL CORE CASES

Stroke
Management of patients with stroke: SIGN guideline.
http://www.sign.ac.uk

RESPIRATORY CORE CASES

Pneumonia
British Thoracic Society (BTS) Guidelines for the Management of Community
Acquired Pneumonia in Adults.
http://www.brit-thoracic.org.uk

Asthma
BTS/SIGN British Guideline on the Management of Asthma.
http://www.brit-thoracic.org.uk

Pulmonary Embolism
BTS Guidelines for the Management of Suspected Acute Pulmonary Embolism.
http://www.brit-thoracic.org.uk

COPD
Chronic Obstructive Pulmonary Disease: NICE guideline.
http://www.nice.org.uk

PAEDIATRIC CORE CASES

Diabetes
Evidence-based guidelines for the management of diabetes in children and young adults. SIGN guideline appraised by Royal College of Paediatrics and Child Health (RCPCH).
http://www.rcpch.ac.uk

OBSTETRIC AND GYNAECOLOGY CORE CASES

Antenatal Care
Antenatal care - routine care for the healthy pregnant woman: Royal College of Obstetrics and Gynaecology (RCOG) guideline.
http://www.rcog.org.uk

Infertility
Fertility: assessment and treatment for people with fertility problems: RCOG guideline.
http://www.rcog.org.uk

Induction of Labour
Induction of Labour: RCOG guideline.
http://www.rcog.org.uk

PASTEST – DEDICATED TO YOUR SUCCESS

PasTest has been publishing books for medical students and doctors for over 30 years. Our extensive experience means that we are always one step ahead when it comes to knowledge of current trends in undergraduate exams.

We use only the best authors, which enables us to tailor our books to meet your revision needs. We incorporate feedback from candidates to ensure that our books are continually improved.

This commitment to quality ensures that students who buy PasTest books achieve successful exam results.

Delivery to your door

With a busy lifestyle, nobody enjoys walking to the shops for something that may or may not be in stock. Let us take the hassle and deliver direct to your door. We will dispatch your book within 24 hours of receiving your order.

How to Order:

www.pastest.co.uk

To order books safely and securely online, shop at our website.

Telephone: +44 (0)1565 752000 Fax: +44 (0)1565 650264

For priority mail order and have your credit card to hand when you call.

Write to us at:

PasTest Ltd
FREEPOST
Haig Road
Parkgate Industrial Estate
Knutsford
WA16 7BR

PASTEST BOOKS FOR MEDICAL STUDENTS

PasTest are the specialists in study guides and revision courses for medical qualifications. For over 30 years we have been helping doctors to achieve their potential. The PasTest range of books for medical students includes:

EMQs for Medical Students Volume 1   1 901198 65 0
Adam Feather et al

EMQs for Medical Students Volume 2   1 901198 69 3
Adam Feather et al

EMQs for Medical Students Volume 3 Practice Papers

          1 904627 07 2

Adam Feather et al

Total Revision: EMQs for Medical Students   1 904627 22 6
Richard Bellamy, Muzlifah Haniffa

Essential MCQs for Medical Finals, Second edition   1 901198 20 0
Rema Wasan, Delilah Hassanally, Balvinder Wasan

Essential MCQs for Surgical Finals, Second edition   1 901198 15 4
Delilah Hassanally, Rema Singh

Essential MCQs in Clinical Pharmacology   1 901198 32 4
Delilah Hassanally, Rema Singh

Essential MCQs in Obstetrics and Gynaecology   1 901198 34 0
Diana Hamilton-Fairley

OSCEs for Medical Students, Volume 1   1 904627 09 9
Adam Feather, Ramanathan Visvanathan, John SP Lumley

OSCEs for Medical Students, Volume 2   1 904627 10 2
Adam Feather, Ramanathan Visvananthan, John SP Lumley

OSCEs for Medical Students, Volume 3   1 904627 11 0
Adam Feather, Ramanathan Visvananthan, John SP Lumley, Jonathan Round